Easy Hikes

CLOSE to
Home

SACRAMENTO

including
Davis, Roseville, and Auburn

JORDAN SUMMERS

MENASHA RIDGE PRESS
Birmingham, Alabama

This book is meant only as a guide to select trails in the Sacramento area and does not guarantee hiker safety in any way—you hike at your own risk. Neither Menasha Ridge Press nor Jordan Summers is liable for property loss or damage, personal injury, or death that result in any way from accessing or hiking the trails described in the following pages. Please be aware that hikers have been injured in the Sacramento area. Be especially cautious when walking on or near boulders, steep inclines, and drop-offs, and do not attempt to explore terrain that may be beyond your abilities. To help ensure an uneventful hike, please read carefully the introduction to this book, and perhaps get further safety information and guidance from other sources. Familiarize yourself thoroughly with the areas you intend to visit before venturing out. Ask questions, and prepare for the unforeseen. Familiarize yourself with current weather reports, maps of the area you intend to visit, and any relevant park regulations.

Copyright © 2009 Jordan Summers
All rights reserved
Printed in the United States of America
Published by Menasha Ridge Press
Distributed by Publishers Group West
First edition, first printing

ISBN 978-0-89732-698-8

Cover by Scott McGrew
Cover photo by Jordan Summers
Text design by Annie Long
Maps by Scott McGrew and Jordan Summers
Interior photos by Jordan Summers

Menasha Ridge Press
P.O. Box 43673
Birmingham, AL 35243
www.menasharidge.com

Contents

About the Author

Jordan Summers

Jordan Summers, a native of
North Carolina, grew up near
the Smoky Mountains of Ten-
nessee and the Blue Ridge
Mountains of Virginia. His teen
years, spent in La Jolla, California, introduced him to new terrain and to the Sierra Club.

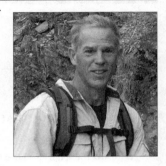

Summers's undergradu-
ate years at the U.S. Air Force
Academy in Colorado exposed
him to even more diverse hiking in the Four Corners region:
desert, canyon, forest, and mountain.

A high-tech career in Southern California brought him
near the mountains for hikes of all kinds—day hikes, ultralight
weekends, or weeklong treks. As friends asked Summers to
arrange and lead trips, it became apparent that he needed to
acquire some new skills. An educational expedition in Wyo-
ming's Wind River Range not only enhanced those skills but
taught Summers how to safely share the outdoor experience
with others, using Leave No Trace techniques.

As his daughter and son grew to become more constant
hiking partners, Summers had to tackle the problem of how to
transport the family's gear into the wilderness. Llamas worked
well at this, as it turned out, and by 1991 Summers was leading
treks with llamas into wilderness areas of Oregon and California. Summers also served during this time as a local chapter
president of the Sierra Club.

Sacramento has been Summers's gateway to the Sierra
Nevada and Coast Range for more than a decade.

Introduction

Welcome to *Easy Hikes Close to Home: Sacramento*. This title in the *Easy Hikes* series is organized according to three Greater Sacramento regions: Urban Hikes; Delta Area Hikes; and Foothills Hikes.

Numbered map icons on the inside front cover locate each primary trailhead and are keyed to the table of contents and narrative text for each trail. On the inside back cover, a map legend defines symbols for parking, restrooms, trail features, and other details. Armed with this handy guidebook, you can quickly head out the door and, well, take a hike!

Overview

Mileage shown for each hike corresponds to the total distance from start to finish, for loops, out-and-backs, figure eights, or a combination of shapes. You can shorten or extend some of the hikes with connecting trails.

Trail Maps

Maps for each hike include GPS coordinates. Based on data downloaded from the author's handheld GPS unit and and plotted onto a digital U.S. Geological Survey (USGS) topo map, the coordinates are shown in two formats: as latitude/longitude and as UTM (Universal Transverse Mercator) coordinates.

HIKING ESSENTIALS

Boots should be your footwear of choice. Sport sandals are popular, but they leave much of your foot exposed and vulnerable to hazardous plants, thorns, rocks, and sharp twigs.

When it comes to water, err on the side of excess. Hydrate prior to your hike, carry (and drink) six ounces of water for every mile you plan to hike, and hydrate after the hike. Pack along a couple of small bottles even for short hikes. You may decide to linger on the trail, or take an alternate route and extend your time outdoors.

Always plan for unpredictable scenarios by carrying these items, in addition to water:

Map	Flashlight with extra batteries
Compass	Rain protection and a sweater or windbreaker, even in warm weather
Basic first-aid supplies, such as Band-Aids and aspirin	
Knife	Sun protection
Windproof matches or a lighter and fire starter	Insect repellent
	Whistle
Snacks	

GENERAL TIPS

The whole point of your outing is to enjoy nature, fresh air, and exercise. Here are a few tips to enhance your excursion:

- Avoid weekends and traditional holidays if possible; otherwise, go early in the morning. Trails that are packed in the summer are often clear during the colder months and during rainy times (but never hike during a thunderstorm).

- Before you hit the trail, double-check your map, and don't set out on the trail until you have the information you need.

- Once on the trail, be careful at overlooks, stay back from the edge of outcrops, and be absolutely sure of your footing wherever you are.

- Hike only on open trails. Respect trail and road closures, avoid trespassing on private land, and obtain permits if required. Leave gates as you found them or as marked.

- Stay on the existing trail, and avoid any littering.

- When hiking with children, use common sense to judge a child's capacity to hike a particular trail, and expect that the child may tire and need to be carried. Make sure children are adequately clothed for the weather, have proper shoes, and are protected from the sun with sunscreen. Kids dehydrate quickly, so make sure you have plenty of fluids for everyone.

- Take your time along the trails, whether you are doing one of this guide's short hikes or hours-long treks. In other words: Don't miss the trees for the forest. You may finish some of the "hike times" long before or after that suggested in the Overview box. A short-distance hike with a lot of up-and-downs may take more time and energy than a longer, flatter hike.

- Participate in online wildlife observation counts. Cornell Lab of Ornithology operates **www.ebird.org** where you can login for free and submit bird lists or find out what people are seeing at some of the area's birding hot spots. A similar count is being done for butterflies at **www.wisconsinbutterflies.org/butterflies/sightings.**

- Never spook animals. An unannounced approach, a sudden movement, or a loud noise startles most animals, and a surprised animal can be dangerous. Give them plenty of space.

- Be courteous to others you encounter on the trails.

- Look up! Keep an eye out for standing dead trees and storm-damaged living trees with loose or broken limbs that can fall at any time.

- Know your ability, and carry necessary supplies for changes in weather or other conditions.

TRAIL RECOMMENDATIONS

Hikes to Rivers and along Creeks

02 Effie Yeaw Nature Center Trails
05 Cosumnes River Preserve Trails
06 Lodi Lake Nature Trail
07 River Bend–Majestic Oaks Loop Trail
08 Grizzly Island Wildlife Area Trail
11 Hidden Falls Trails
12 Lake Clementine Trail
13 Confluence Trail
14 Robie Point Firebreak Trail
16 Independence Trail: West Branch
17 Buttermilk Bend Trail

Hikes with Old Growth Trees

09 Indian Grinding Rock Loop Trails

Lake Hikes

04 Davis–Covell Greenbelt
05 Cosumnes River Preserve Trails
06 Lodi Lake Nature Trail
10 Avery's Pond Trail
12 Lake Clementine Trail

Hikes Good for Runners

01 Capitol Park Loop
02 Effie Yeaw Nature Center Trails
04 Davis–Covell Greenbelt
11 Hidden Falls Trails
12 Lake Clementine Trail
13 Confluence Trail
14 Robie Point Firebreak Trail

15 Hardrock Trail
16 Independence Trail: West Branch

Hikes with Dogs

01 Capitol Park Loop
04 Davis–Covell Greenbelt
11 Hidden Falls Trails
12 Lake Clementine Trail
13 Confluence Trail
14 Robie Point Firebreak Trail

Hikes with Historic Sites or Relics

22 Indian Grinding Rock Loop Trails
12 Lake Clementine Trail
15 Hardrock Trail
16 Independence Trail: West Branch

Waterfall and Cascades Hikes

11 Hidden Falls Trails
12 Lake Clementine Trail

Wheelchair Accessible

01 Capitol Park Loop
02 Effie Yeaw Nature Center Trails
03 UC Davis Arboretum Trail
04 Davis–Covell Greenbelt
05 Cosumnes River Preserve Trails
06 Lodi Lake Nature Trail
07 River Bend–Majestic Oaks Loop Trail
09 Indian Grinding Rock Loop Trails
11 Hidden Falls Trails
16 Independence Trail: West Branch

Wildlife Hikes

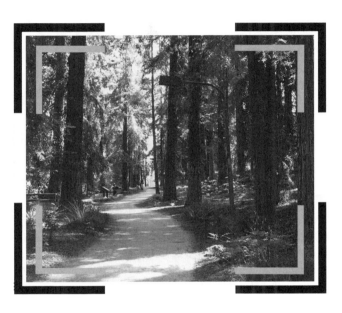

Urban Hikes

01 Capitol Park Loop

■ OVERVIEW

LENGTH: 1.5 miles	**ACCESS:** No fees or permits
CONFIGURATION: Loop	**MAPS:** USGS Sacramento East; park-brochure map
WATER REQUIRED: 1 liter	
SCENERY: Arboretum, statuary, monuments, memorials	**WHEELCHAIR TRAVERSABLE:** Yes, if you access trail at 11th and L streets
EXPOSURE: Some sun, some shade	**FACILITIES:** On- and off-street parking; water fountains; benches
TRAFFIC: Moderate	**DRIVING DISTANCE:** 1 mile
TRAIL SURFACE: Paved walkways	**SPECIAL COMMENTS:** This route can be walked in any direction, depending on the interests of the hiker or location of your parking space.
HIKING TIME: 2 hours	
SEASON: Year-round	

■ SNAPSHOT

The California State Capitol Park is one of the most outstanding capitol grounds to be found in any state. You can meander aimlessly through the dozen or so memorials, which are spread among hundreds of trees, bushes, and flowers from around the world in this 40-acre Victorian-style garden.

■ CLOSE-UP

Capitol Park can be accessed from any point along its 12-city-block length, and so it seems natural to start closest to where you park. The starting point of this hike is on the north side steps at 11th Street. You can get a pamphlet at the State Capitol Museum, which offers a good map and an informative description of the park's many features.

Several major plantings, or "beautifications," were undertaken between the park's inception in 1869 and the most recent beautification in 1951, when the capitol annex was built. Rather than plantings having been added to the park, only memorials

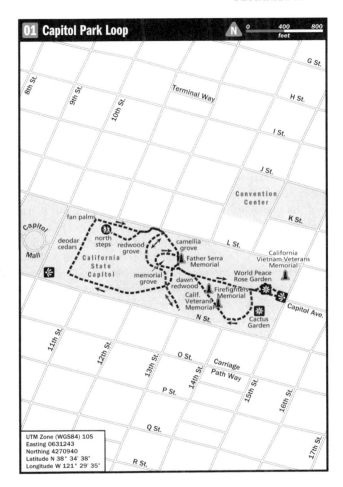

UTM Zone (WGS84) 10S
Easting 0631243
Northing 4270940
Latitude N 38° 34' 38"
Longitude W 121° 29' 35"

have been erected since the 1950s. Some of the oldest trees, the "heritage" plantings, have succumbed to age or storms.

The sidewalks that encircle the park are lined with palms, and trees line the walkways throughout the park; both paths are designed for the easiest and most complete access to the park's features. Paths are not always at right angles, so the park has a very natural appearance.

There is no one specific direction for visitors to travel through this park. If you turn right from the starting point, you will see a line of coast redwoods, original plantings from an 1872 beautification. A grove of coast redwood and giant sequoia is planted on the north side of the capitol, just to the east of the security entrance. One of the trees in this grove is called the "moon tree" by park staff because its seed was carried on an Apollo lunar mission and then planted on its return. The tree is not signed, however.

As you angle toward L Street, you will see the sole Italian stone pine remaining from the original planting in 1872. Turn right at 12th Street and head to the east entrance of the capitol, where you have some excellent photo opportunities. From here, walk east on the central promenade, where memorials and commemorative gardens are on either side of you.

Next, walk to the 15th Street end of the park, where you will have some excellent photo opportunities of the capitol. The World Peace Rose Garden features a fragrant and colorful garden with benches dedicated by notable women who are themselves dedicated to peace.

The California Vietnam Veterans Memorial is adjacent to the rose garden. Its striking theme features stylized ammunition and starkly contrasting white limestone that holds black granite panels bearing the names of missing or dead California veterans of that war. The inside of the circular monument features reliefs and sculptures representing various aspects of Americans' armed service in Southeast Asia. The centerpiece of the memorial is a life-size bronze statue of a 19-year-old soldier. The Firefighters Memorial is also made of granite and bronze and dramatically depicts the dangers facing firefighters in action. These two sculptures were added in 2002. Out toward

N Street is the California Veterans Memorial, which is dedicated to all Californians who have served in the armed forces. Its use of photography and stone is unique.

An Indian grinding rock is to the west before you reach another coast redwood–giant sequoia grove with a comfortable bench encouraging rest and contemplation. Make your way north again, where the Spanish-American War Memorial, the Civil War Memorial, and the Liberty Bell Memorial are grouped among flowers and trees. An example of the dawn redwood, the only deciduous redwood species, is here. From the interior of China, this tree was long thought to be extinct.

A life-size monument featuring Father Junipero Serra is prominently featured in front of the colorful camellia grove. Standing beneath a lamppost shaped like a shepherd's crook, Father Serra's bronze statue looks down on a bronze relief map of California mounted on a black marble pedestal.

You can wander around the inside perimeter sidewalk on the west side of the capitol, where a row of deodar cedars flanks the walkway for two city blocks. The corner is a good spot from which to take some pictures.

Walking along these pathways on a weekend morning is a real pleasure at Capitol Park, where you can find both natural and man-made art. The architecture is classic and unimposing. The gardens and groves, with their thousands of flowers, bushes, and trees, are just waiting for you to view, smell, touch, photograph, and wander.

■ TO THE TRAILHEAD

From Interstate 5 North in downtown Sacramento, exit at J Street and drive 12 blocks to 15th Street, where you will turn right. Drive two blocks to L Street and take another right. Parking is available at metered spaces on L Street. Or drive to Ninth Street, turn left, and make another left on N Street, where there is more metered parking. There are also several covered garages nearby.

■ OVERVIEW

LENGTH: 0.75–2.5 miles

CONFIGURATION: 3 loop trails

WATER REQUIRED: 1 liter

SCENERY: Riparian zone along American River

EXPOSURE: Shaded along 75% of trail

TRAFFIC: Varied, depending on the day of the week

TRAIL SURFACE: Pebble and duff; river cobble and sand

HIKING TIME: 0.5–2 hours

SEASON: Open November–January, 9:30 a.m.–4 p.m.; February–October, 9 a.m.–5 p.m.; closed Thanksgiving, Christmas Day, and New Year's Day

ACCESS: No fees or permits

MAPS: USGS Carmichael; maps of the nature trails are available online and at the nature center.

FACILITIES: Restrooms, picnic tables, outdoor theater, gift shop

WHEELCHAIR TRAVERSABLE: Yes, from the parking lot up to the nature center and possibly along parts of River History Trail. Trails are bumpy, slippery, and muddy in spots.

DRIVING DISTANCE: 7 miles

SPECIAL COMMENTS: The Effie Yeaw Nature Center (inside Ancil Hoffman County Park, 2850 San Lorenzo Way, Carmichael, California; [916] 489-4918) offers programs for all ages every Saturday and Sunday at 1:30 p.m. Visit the center's Web site, www.effieyeaw.org, for details, a calendar, and maps.

■ SNAPSHOT

This 77-acre nature preserve offers a glimpse of the once-vast riparian and oak woodlands, shrublands, meadows, and aquatic habitats along the American River. Deer, squirrels, wild turkeys, rabbits, snakes, hawks, owls, woodpeckers, songbirds, and waterfowl add to the adventure of the three self-guided walking trails.

■ CLOSE-UP

The Effie Yeaw Nature Center captures a time when Maidu Nisenan people camped along this area each summer, enjoying the plentiful food in this riparian habitat that once extended 5 miles on either side of the American River. Deer, rabbit, squirrel, fox, turkey, fowl, crayfish, and salmon, and plentiful valley oaks,

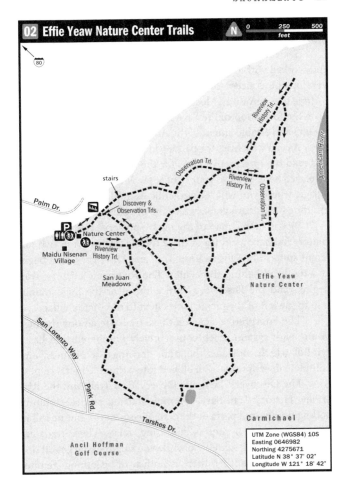

02 Effie Yeaw Nature Center Trails

N   0   250   500
feet

Riverview History Trl.

American River

Observation Trl.

stairs

Riverview History Trl.

Observation Trl.

Palm Dr.

Discovery & Observation Trls.

P

Nature Center

Maidu Nisenan Village

Riverview History Trl.

San Juan Meadows

Effie Yeaw Nature Center

San Lorenzo Way

Park Rd.

Tarshes Dr.

Carmichael

Ancil Hoffman Golf Course

| UTM Zone (WGS84) 10S |
| Easting 0646982 |
| Northing 4275671 |
| Latitude N 38° 37' 02" |
| Longitude W 121° 18' 42" |

willows, sedges, and reeds—all of the essential ingredients for Native American life—could be found where you now walk.

In the 1950s and 1960s, Effie Yeaw—a teacher, conservationist, and environmental educator—began leading natural and cultural history walks in this area formerly known as Deterding Woods.

Yeaw raised interest in preserving the lands along the river and worked with the Sacramento County Parks Department to develop the concept of a parkway along the river that would include these grounds. Most importantly, her vision helped stimulate the formation of the Save the American River Association (SARA) and establishment of the American River Parkway.

As you walk from the parking lot to the nature center, pause and read the interpretive signs for the native California species displayed here. Look to your right at the Maidu Nisenan summer village, where you will see authentic examples of a tule shelter, grinding rock, acorn granary, and fire pit, plus a shade shelter.

Pick up a free map of the nature preserve trails inside the center. You have a choice of three trails, which start in two different spots: The Observation Trail and Discovery Trail begin at a trailhead behind the center. The Riverview History Trail begins (and the Discovery Trail ends) near the huge walnut tree to the left of the picnic tables next to the Maidu village.

The interpretive signs on these trails are among the best in any park system. Each consecutively numbered sign has a symbol which indicates the trail, drawings or pictures, and complete descriptions—all etched into a durable metal sign.

The Discovery Trail, the Observation Trail, and the Riverview History Trail have common starting points, common ending points, and parts of the trail in common—but not all in the same way. If it sounds confusing, relax. These trails are delightful and well signed. So while you might easily get off one route and onto another, there is no fear of becoming "temporarily mislocated."

Step back out of the nature center, turn left, and walk around the building. Pass the Himalayan blackberries on your right, then pass the small outdoor theater, and your trailhead is another ten feet.

This is a dual trailhead—straight ahead for the Observation Trail and right for the Discovery Trail. The Observation

Trail both starts and ends here. The Discovery Trail starts here but ends at the start of the Riverview History Trail.

Ahead, on the Observation Trail, you will start out with a nicely shaded, winding, duff-covered trail that leads to a bench atop the only stairs on the trails. Look at the moss covering the north side of the trees in this damp valley-oak grove. Momentarily, the trail will open up and join the Riverview History Trail for a brief bit of full sunshine. In this open area, the native grasses and sedges proliferated after floods.

Pay close attention as you approach the river. The Observation Trail makes a turn to the right, and the Riverview History Trail turns to the left ten feet farther along. Take the Observation Trail, heading south on this duff trail and ignoring the first trail that comes in from the right. Although that trail from the right will reconnect with this trail and lead back to the center, the Observation Trail continues ahead. Look to the left at the moonscape of large river cobble and boulders. This spectacular scene is just part of the original land granted to John Sutter.

Make a right onto the next trail and plunge into a thick copse of live oak, where you can feel the air temperature drop. Sample more blackberries if there are any. The undergrowth is so lush and the foliage so thick that it is difficult to hear or see others, which affords a nice sense of solitude. Take a break at the bench where the trail turns briefly north.

A small meadow ringed by live oak offers a nice spot for deer to browse. The trail crosses Riverview History Trail but soon turns toward the nature center, so do not let the deer capture your attention at this junction. A short uphill section returns you to the trailhead and the start of Discovery Trail.

On Discovery Trail, you will descend gently alongside Himalayan blackberries, past giant—fallen and decomposing—valley oak, alongside Dutchman's pipevine, all of which provides habitat for beetles, ground squirrels, hummingbirds, and woodpeckers.

As you look to your right, you may see deer lounging near the trail and around the margin of San Juan Meadows.

The meadow is defined by huge valley oaks. These prototypically spreading oaks are found only in California and are the largest species of oak in North America. Deer and rabbit are plentiful here, and the opportunities for outstanding wildlife photos are abundant. But stay on the trails—particularly in this area. As in most parks, this one posts cautions about poison oak and even has interpretive signs pointing it out along this section of the trail.

Turkeys are abundant in this area and you will notice their signs everywhere if you do not slip on or trip over them first. And they roost in trees! Enjoy the sandy, winding trail as you read the signs on the way to the nature pond. A clean bench there makes a great perch to observe bugs, reptiles, and birds.

After winding through sedge-filled groves of live oak and western redbud, the trail begins to turn to sand and river cobble. At the junction with the Riverview History Trail, turn left. Walk past your initial crossing with this trail and head west along the San Juan Meadows. The Discovery Trail ends where the Riverview History Trail begins—at the huge, two-toned walnut tree.

Now you are at the beginning of the Riverview History Trail, which you have seen and crossed several times. The trail, made of river cobble and sand, is partly service road and is therefore potholed in spots. On this, the most openly exposed of all the trails, walk straight; the trails you walked earlier cross your path. You will angle toward the American River. Beautiful modern homes on the cliffs above you stand in stark contrast to the quiet as you approach the river. You will take a much smaller footpath off to the right, angling another 50 feet toward the river. If you happen to miss this turn, you will find a bench about 100 feet ahead. Turn there and come back to this trail alongside the river.

Head south along the trail and try to imagine the view without the aftermath of gold dredging. A bench ahead on your right is a great spot for that and for bird watching.

At the next signed junction to the right, you will turn and retrace your steps from the Observation Trail as the Riverview History Trail now joins with it for the return to the nature center.

■ MORE FUN

Folsom State Recreation Area has a 90-mile network of multiuse trails that includes the Pioneer Express Trail as well as a 21-mile segment of the American Discovery Trail, the nation's first coast-to-coast nonmotorized recreation trail.

■ TO THE TRAILHEAD

From downtown Sacramento, take US 50 east 5 miles to the Watt Avenue North exit. Follow Watt Avenue north 0.8 miles to Fair Oaks Avenue. Turn right on Fair Oaks and drive 4 miles to Van Alstine (El Camino to the left). Turn right on Van Alstine and in 0.3 miles, turn left on California. Go 0.2 miles to Tarshes Drive, where you will turn right at the Ancil Hoffman Park sign. Drive 0.4 miles along Tarshes Drive to the entrance kiosk and then 0.2 miles to San Lorenzo Way; then turn left and head 0.1 mile to the nature center parking lot. The trailheads are on either side of the nature center.

03 UC Davis Arboretum Trail

■ OVERVIEW

LENGTH: 3.5 miles	**ACCESS:** No fees or permits
CONFIGURATION: Loop	**MAPS:** USGS Merritt, Davis
WATER REQUIRED: 1 liter	**WHEELCHAIR TRAVERSABLE:** Yes
SCENERY: Flora from around the world	**FACILITIES:** Water fountains and restrooms in various locations near the trail. See UC Davis Arboretum map for exact locations.
EXPOSURE: Mostly shaded	
TRAFFIC: Light	
TRAIL SURFACE: Asphalt, pebble, and sand	**DRIVING DISTANCE:** 14 miles
HIKING TIME: 2 hours, plus lingering time	**SPECIAL COMMENTS:** This hike is not only beautiful and enjoyable but accessible and educational, too.
SEASON: Year-round	

■ SNAPSHOT

More than 4,000 plants and flowers are on display at the University of California, Davis, Arboretum in 18 collections and gardens. If you want to learn about the flora in California's biozones, a few hours among these magnificent gardens and collections will satisfy your interest.

■ CLOSE-UP

The UC Davis Arboretum Trail winds peacefully along an interstate highway and city streets. On this hike, you start out by walking southwest through fragrant lavender, rosemary, and other herbs growing on both sides of the Mediterranean Collection along Putah Creek Lagoon.

When Putah Creek's channel was diverted in the 1870s, what remained was this abandoned oxbow—the old north channel—which dried up over the years and became the sole depression among otherwise flat farmland. From its beginnings as an actual farm for horticultural instruction in World War I

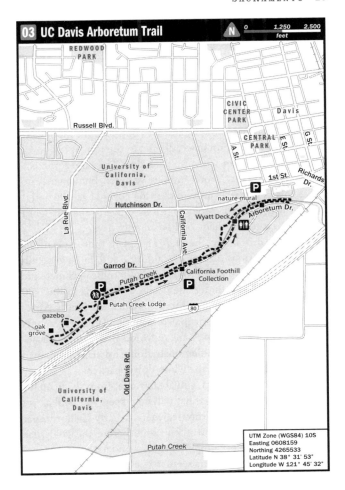

until 1936, the arboretum area became the collection point
for an abundance of unwanted materials. The arboretum
was founded February 29 of that same year, when students, fac-
ulty, and administrators joined in their traditional "leap day

campus-improvement project." This included the arboretum's "first planting," which comprised many of the trees seen along the south shore from Wyatt Deck to the California Avenue Bridge.

The design and placement of the arboretum included plants native to California that have low water requirements, and protected the magnificent 400-year-old valley oaks (*Quercus lobata*) growing in the California Foothill Collection. Caretakers of the arboretum have adhered to the principle of using the natural landform whenever possible. The larger ponds at the south end of the arboretum were sculpted, but you may not notice this as you walk around the vine-covered gazebo and its fragrant white-flower garden. The oak grove to the far right is popular for catching shade on hot summer days.

The plants lining the trail represent those specifically native to the various regions of California and, more generally, to the regions of the world where a Mediterranean climate predominates. You will find gardens and collections in this 100-acre arboretum that represent areas such as South Africa, Australia, or South America; also, specific plants are grouped by type, as in the oak groves, the redwood grove, and the acacia collection, and there are demonstration gardens and horticultural theme gardens, like the white-flower garden.

As you might expect, you are never far from shade on this trail, but a broad-brimmed hat will help keep you cool as you browse around at the boathouse, where an early-California garden displays plants found in the state before the gold rush. There really are no empty spaces—understory trees and bushes, grasses, and flowers seem to occupy the terrain and line the creekside path.

Pass to the right of Putah Creek Lodge, with its inviting fire pit and seating area, through the South American Collection with its lush Cuyamaca cypress, and then into the dense, cool shade of the acacia grove. As you walk around the little side trails and groves, take notice of the soil underfoot on these bordered trails. The silt and plant debris deposited alongside this former channel were the ingredients that created the rich sandy loam that is so beneficial to all of the plants here. Towering Torrey pines and spreading California sycamore suddenly dwarf any understory plants, but California poppies can be counted on for color.

There are very few surprising turns on this trail, and all are clearly marked. Aleppo pine, buckeye, and California box elder lead into the valley-oak grove as you head toward the Mondavi Center for the Performing Arts. The California Foothill Collection features live oak, toyon, mesa oak, gray pine, and a streamside covered with wild grapes, in addition to a five-foot-diameter valley oak.

Flowers and shrubs accompany you past Marak Hall Drive, and native Californian plants fill the side gardens just ahead of Wyatt Deck and the redwood grove. California fuchsia, dwarf coyote bush, Torrey pine and Santa Cruz ironwood, Catalina Island mountain mahogany, Canary Island pine and sand mesa manzanita, shooting star, and penstemon are all part of this impressively colorful display.

Leap Day 1941 saw the planting of the redwood trees in this grove. Because they are not native to the valley, these coast redwoods were hand-watered by energetic students, who are responsible for the trees' maturing into the grove you see today. This is the spot to stop and take notes and pictures and have a drink or a snack. The picnic tables offer solitude within these giant trees.

Art and nature are as important as the gardens to the arboretum. The huge, colorful, and oversize nature lesson that is found in the tunnel-wall mural is an example of that partnership. Take the left fork after this tunnel and enter the Australian collection. Your turnaround takes you to the other side of the creek, onto a dirt path just opposite the mural tunnel. Meander through the North Coast Collection opposite the redwood grove. Your dirt path will return to asphalt at the next footbridge. Formosan redwood, soquel coast redwood, and egg-shaped sculptures precede the desert collection, with its sunny patch of blossoming prickly-pear cactus and looming agave plant.

Gray pine, Oaxaca pine, Chinese juniper, and a long line of redbud lead into the South American Collection and back to the trailhead.

■ MORE FUN

Group tours can be arranged with 30 days' notice by calling (530) 752-4880.

■ TO THE TRAILHEAD

From Interstate 5 in downtown Sacramento, drive 13 miles west on I-80 to Davis. Exit I-80 at UC Davis (Exit 71), and turn right on Old Davis Road. Continue straight ahead onto California Avenue and make the next left onto La Rue Road. Turn left on Putah Creek Lodge Road and then right into the parking area. Parking is also available in Lots 47 and 48 on La Rue Road and costs $6; you can use a credit card or $1 bills. Parking is limited on weekdays, but on weekends it is free and more broadly available. The trail described here starts at the Putah Creek Lodge footbridge. You can begin your hike from any point along the path, but this hike begins at the Mediterranean Collection at the footbridge on the side of the creek opposite the Putah Creek Lodge.

■ OVERVIEW

LENGTH: 2.7 miles	**SEASON:** Year-round
CONFIGURATION: Loop	**ACCESS:** No fees or permits
WATER REQUIRED: 0.5 liters	**MAPS:** USGS Davis, Merritt
SCENERY: Urban green space with wildlife-viewing platforms	**FACILITIES:** Restrooms here and at Northstar Park
EXPOSURE: Plenty of sun and shade	**WHEELCHAIR TRAVERSABLE:** Yes
TRAFFIC: Moderate but not crowded	**DRIVING DISTANCE:** 15 miles
TRAIL SURFACE: Asphalt pavement	**SPECIAL COMMENTS:** This hike features playgrounds, lawn sculptures, and a nature walk.
HIKING TIME: 1.5 hours	

■ SNAPSHOT

The Davis–Covell Greenbelt links the Davis Community Park and Northstar Park while it weaves through neighborhoods and their playgrounds. The well-lit asphalt path has location signs and easy access to all the adjacent communities.

■ CLOSE-UP

The Davis–Covell Greenbelt is a wonderful path to walk and includes a surprising diversity of interesting sights. The described hike begins at the pedestrian overpass at the north end of the Davis Community Park. There is an alternative starting point, also with parking and restrooms, at Northstar Park, which is located at the north end of the greenbelt. If you are arriving on foot, almost every side street along the path accesses the greenbelt, which winds through the surrounding communities.

Once across the bridge, the trail splits at the first playground. You will be returning along the path to the left. Walk straight, generally north northwest, along the greenbelt as it

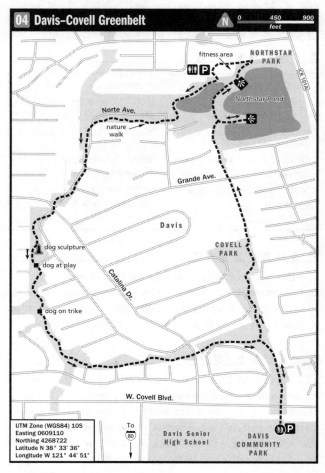

To 80

meanders through Covell Park. The names of the streets you pass all have a Spanish theme, and nearly every street has an entrance to the greenbelt. Within the first half mile, you will see tennis courts, benches, barbecue grills, swings, slides, merry-go-rounds, and other leisure amenities.

Continue past the empty field to your left and cross Grande Avenue. A fence to your right marks the border of the Northstar Park wetland area. A variety of waterfowl inhabit this small pond, and, from the sounds of it, so does a bevy of frogs. A nicely designed viewing platform extends into the wetland, allowing you to observe the wildlife. Egrets, herons, Canada geese, mallards, and coots comprise just a partial list of birds that live or visit here. An identically designed, but much smaller, viewpoint is located just 500 feet down the path on these tiny, wooded islands.

Pass the aerating pond to the left of the path and walk toward Anderson Road, where you will turn left. A fitness and warm-up area sits on the path's left just 100 feet past the smaller viewpoint. This is a good reason for beginning an exercise run at the Northstar Park and using the parking lot on the west side of the Tandem Properties building.

Continuing on the described path takes you through the parking lot, past the restrooms on the left, southward toward your trailhead. You will once again pass the aerating pond, with the playing fields of Northstar Park to your right.

There is a nature walk on your right just after the playing fields. An informational kiosk lists a huge variety of trees, shrubs, and flowers to be found here and also along the path. Walk west along the gravel path through the shady nature area and make sure to look up as you pass under the welded arbors.

Exiting the nature walk, turn to the south again along this pleasant path. Within a few minutes, you will cross Catalina Drive and reach another of the small parks along the walk. Eucalyptus trees tower over the path as you enter Greenbelt Area #10. You may not have expected artwork to be among the interesting things you would be seeing on this walk. Rendered in bronze and natural stone, several clever installations liven the pathway. Keep a lookout for a turkey-chasing dog here. As you pass Ecuador Place, you may notice another friendly dog ready to share his water with your pup. And as you watch out for bicycles along the path, be on the alert for happy tricycle riders around Estrella Place.

The route described here continues straight south. If you want to wander farther west, turn right and walk through the tunnel under Anderson Road when the trail ends, and just one block farther west you can pick up an alternate trail back to the north. Your path continues through signed greenbelt areas with playgrounds, Frisbee fields, picnic tables, and benches before crossing Catalina Drive and reentering Covell Park to the east. At the playground, you will take the path to the right and head toward the pedestrian overpass where you began your walk.

■ MORE FUN

Before you get on the interstate, stop in for a burger at Redrum Burgers, at the intersection of Olive Drive and Russell Boulevard. When Murder Burger, a straightforward burger-and-beer joint expanded to Rocklin, residents objected to the violent nature of the name, and so a renaming contest was held wherein Redrum was conceived. It continues to be known for its wide variety of beers and low-fat-beef burgers (ask about the Zoom).

■ TO THE TRAILHEAD

From Interstate 5 in downtown Sacramento, drive west on I-80 to the Russell Boulevard exit in Davis. Follow Russell Boulevard under the railroad overpass and bear slightly right at First Street, where Russell Boulevard becomes E Street. Turn right at Fourth Street and then left on F Street, one block later. Continue north on F Street ten blocks to West Covell Boulevard. Turn left on West Covell Boulevard and then left into the parking lot just before the pedestrian overpass. Your trailhead is at the end of the overpass.

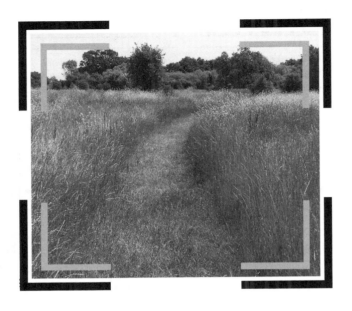

Delta Area Hikes

05 Cosumnes River Preserve Trails

■ OVERVIEW

LENGTH: 4.1 miles	**ACCESS:** No fees or permits
CONFIGURATION: Connected loops	**MAPS:** USGS Bruceville
WATER REQUIRED: 0.5 liters	**FACILITIES:** Pit toilets in the parking
SCENERY: Open savanna and riparian woodland	lots on both sides of Franklin Road
	SPECIAL COMMENTS: Excellent hands-on displays are included in the visitor center exhibits.
EXPOSURE: Bright in the meadows	
TRAFFIC: Light	
TRAIL SURFACE: Grass or dirt trail; concrete sidewalk	**WHEELCHAIR TRAVERSABLE:** Yes; the Wetlands Trail is a level sidewalk with observation platforms.
HIKING TIME: 2 hours	**DRIVING DISTANCE:** 22 miles
SEASON: Year-round, sunrise–sunset	

■ SNAPSHOT

The River and Wetlands Walks at the Cosumnes River Preserve showcase the plant and wildlife communities of the largest free-flowing river entering the Great Central Valley. Close to town and accessible to all, these trails offer tranquility, beauty, and a sense of what the area once looked like to settlers.

■ CLOSE-UP

The trails at the preserve guide hikers through two of the Central Valley's diminishing plant communities. Here, hikers can stroll through a riparian forest, past a freshwater marsh and vernal pools, and along annual grasslands at a leisurely pace.

The Cosumnes River Preserve is managed by the Nature Conservancy, the U.S. Bureau of Land Management, Ducks Unlimited, the California Department of Fish and Game, the State Lands Commission, the California Department of Water Resources, Sacramento County, and private landowners.

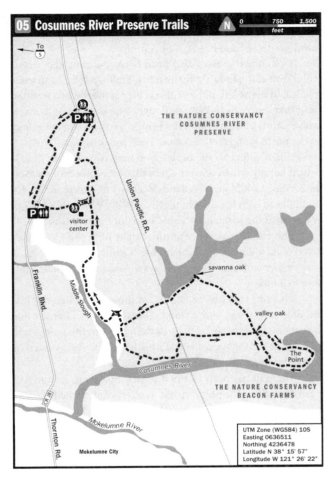

05 Cosumnes River Preserve Trails

N   0   750   1,500
feet

To 5

THE NATURE CONSERVANCY
COSUMNES RIVER
PRESERVE

Union Pacific R.R.

visitor
center

savanna oak

valley oak

Franklin Blvd.

Middle Slough

The
Point

Cosumnes River

THE NATURE CONSERVANCY
BEACON FARMS

CR 13

Thornton Rd.

Mokelumne River

Mokelumne City

UTM Zone (WGS84) 10S
Easting 0636511
Northing 4236478
Latitude N 38° 15' 57"
Longitude W 121° 26' 22"

If your party includes children, the visitor center should be your first stop: let them acquaint themselves with the plants and wildlife they are about to see. Hands-on displays encourage everyone to touch, feel, and learn about the elements of this unique and diminishing environment. Pick up trail maps and interpretive information for the area. The visitor center is staffed by volunteers, who also conduct guided tours. Call ahead for details and hours of operation.

The annual grasses and flowers surrounding the visitor center hint at the flora along the trails. Trailheads for both trails are located to the left of the visitor center at the top of a wooden ramp that descends to Willow Slough. The benches and observation points at each end of the bridge are nice spots to reflect on the posted interpretive material and touch-signs.

When you cross the bridge, you have two choices. One is to turn left onto the concrete sidewalk of the Lost Slough Wetlands Walk. Lost Slough Wetlands Walk is 1 mile long and shares the trailhead with the Cosumnes River Walk. Wetlands Walk can be started at the parking lot across Franklin Boulevard as well.

The trail described here turns right onto the Cosumnes River Walk, following its dirt path south along Middle Slough. A warning sign at the trail's start relates the danger mountain lions pose to humans.

This dirt trail can be flooded at times, but when dry it is smooth, soft, wide, and shaded. Himalayan blackberries line the path on the left, and songbirds exercise both their lungs and their wings. Flashes of color and whistles follow you as you pass by each of the interpretive-sign markers.

The trail has been planned so that hikers are treated to a bit of everything the preserve has to offer. Well marked at every turn, the path even allows for whimsical side trips or loops to allow you see all its features.

The marshland to the east of the trail was restored through the efforts of Ducks Unlimited. Mallard ducks and egrets, redwing blackbirds, and even slow pond turtles move among the tall grasses and reeds. Make a left turn and head to the footbridge on the marsh's south side. Another 200 feet along, head up the wooden step to your right.

A boulevard of majestic valley oaks shades your way as you walk toward the river to the south and then head east, listening to acorn woodpeckers. These beautiful trees shaded the Miwok people, who used the Santa Barbara sedges as material for their intricate baskets, which they used to cook the oaks' abundant acorns.

The scent of the wild California rose becomes stronger as you approach the Cosumnes 0.5 miles above its mouth at the Mokelumne River. The Cosumnes flows about 80 miles from its source high in the El Dorado National Forest to join the Sacramento–San Joaquin Delta. The river and sloughs here are subject to the same tidal forces as those in the San Francisco Bay. These are the spawning grounds of Chinook salmon, and are home to muskrat, beaver, mink, and river otter.

Now it's time to turn north before passing under the railroad trestle. A pair of interpretive signs tells of the work involved in identifying and managing nonnative species. Your grassy trail is exposed as you parallel the Union Pacific tracks. As soon as you turn under the tracks, you will see that the extra sun is worth it.

Immense valley oaks are the highlight of this grassland savanna. The color surrounding you depends on the season, but the lush grasses, wildflowers, and oaks are a backdrop for wonderful memories.

Continue walking east across this vast meadow. At the next trail crossing, you may turn right or go straight, as this route describes. The nesting boxes in the trees are for wood ducks. Kites soaring and spotted towhees scrambling underfoot are hints of the 200 identified species of birds that visit or live here. House finches and sandhill cranes, swans, ducks, geese, and coots flock to this wetland annually.

Complete this mini-loop by walking south and west past The Point, where you may enjoy a rest on the benches placed here as part of a Boy Scout project. Then it's on to a lonesome live oak, where you will turn left and head northwest to the oak-marked junction you passed earlier.

Continue northwest across the meadow toward a grand savanna oak at the edge of a tule marsh. Linger in the shade here and take a moment to use your binoculars while under cover. You won't have to wait long to observe several species from this cool spot.

Now head southwest to follow the trail signs under the tracks and across an old doubletrack, and then make a right at the wooden stairs that you ascended previously. Cross the bridge, turn left, and follow the path back to the visitor center.

When you reach the concrete sidewalk, you have traveled 3.1 miles. The Lost Slough Wetlands Walk is 1 mile long. Within 200 feet, an observation point and benches entice you to rest. The trail continues to the right, past the native ryegrasses.

After crossing the bridge, you will see the uniform growth of the grove of valley oaks planted as acorns in 1988. Brush your hand lightly across the fennel growing here to release more of its fragrant scent as you pass. Butterflies blanket this and other blossoms along the path.

An observation point is conveniently located along the slough just before the trail crosses the road. Another viewing area extends from the parking lot into the wetland on the other side of Franklin Boulevard. There are interpretive signs in the parking lot. The ponds to your right are wet year-round, although they grow and shrink. Another observation deck awaits at the southernmost end of this section of the walk. Cross Franklin Boulevard to return to the visitor center.

■ TO THE TRAILHEAD

From Interstate 5 in Sacramento, drive south 20 miles to the Twin Cities Road exit. Turn east, driving 1 mile to make a right onto Franklin Boulevard south. In 0.4 miles, you will see the Cosumnes River Preserve sign on the right. The visitor center is located on the left, another 1.2 miles down Franklin Boulevard. The trailheads are located next to the visitor center on the left.

■ OVERVIEW

LENGTH: 2.5 miles

CONFIGURATION: Loops

WATER REQUIRED: 0.5 liters

SCENERY: Riparian area with views of the Mokelumne River

EXPOSURE: Shaded trail; little exposure

TRAFFIC: Light on weekday afternoons

TRAIL SURFACE: Asphalt and packed dirt

HIKING TIME: 1.5 hours

SEASON: Year-round, sunrise–sunset

ACCESS: $5 fee

MAPS: USGS Lodi North

FACILITIES: Restrooms near swimming area, outdoor theater

WHEELCHAIR TRAVERSABLE: Yes, on the paved nature trail

DRIVING DISTANCE: 34 miles

SPECIAL COMMENTS: Docent-guided tours can be arranged by contacting Lodi Lake Park, 1101 West Turner Road, Lodi, CA, 95242, (209) 333-6742. Bicycles are not allowed on the trails, and dogs must be leashed. Your canine hiking partner may appreciate a run at the dog fields near the swimming area.

■ SNAPSHOT

The nature trail joins the exercise trail to form a pleasant loop that lets hikers experience the wonderful sights, sounds, and scents to be found in the Mokelumne River riparian area.

■ CLOSE-UP

Rarely does a small town take such care to preserve an important ecological area like the city of Lodi has done with this 58-acre nature area. You know this place is special as soon as you see the murals at the trailhead. Walk straight ahead on the asphalt-paved pathway, the Nature Trail, which will take you generally northeast 0.5 miles. In fact, you could turn around at that point, satisfied that you have seen most of what the park has to offer; but this hike continues on the exercise trail to make a loop around the park and along the former river channel.

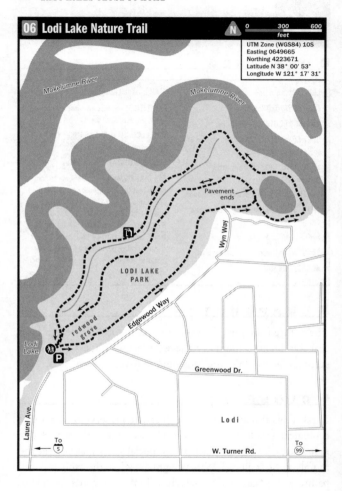

Walk past the outdoor theater set amid a grove of majestic coast redwoods. They may be the most obvious of the trees that are not native to the Central Valley, but they are not the only nonnative species. The Himalayan blackberry (not a foreign handheld device) and black locust (not an insect) are also introduced species that have adapted well to the sandy loam of the valley's riparian environment.

The grasslands that you soon pass display both native and nonnative species. There are informational placards in the ground that have suffered some flood damage, but are generally well placed. Markers attached to the trees seem to last longer.

Valley oaks stand like huge, ponderous ancestors of the area, but even they look up to the noisy foliage of the cotton-woods. When the explorer John C. Fremont came through this area in 1844, he made special comment on the musical rustlings of the leaves of the cottonwoods and oaks. Just about the time you are thinking about relaxing while listening to the trees yourself, nice benches will start appearing like poppies.

Casual trails lead off to the water's edge or across the area between trails, but the Nature Trail continues on the pavement until a substantial, yellow metal post. Continue past the post and your dirt-and-duff trail will lead left around a small pond, which is excellent for spotting frogs, turtles, mallards, and wood ducks amid the dozens of birds hiding in the understory and sprinting along the pond's edge. As you exit the pond area, you will walk past the tree dedicated to the anonymous "E"— perhaps indicating an invitation to eat the mountain of black-berries found here.

The cattails and their resident frogs line the trail as it traces a small creek formed by river water that has soaked the ground. Hummingbirds and a variety of understory-dwelling songbirds and dozens of little brown birds join the frogs just after you pass the viewing platform.

Back at the trailhead, this half of the trail and loop has covered about 1.5 miles. If you want, continue around to the other half of the exercise trail and walk with the outdoor the-ater and redwood grove on your left. There is some exposure here, where your trail runs close to the neighborhood. The unexpected feature of this hike is not that it is so quiet along the trail, but that it is so noisy—with sounds of the trees, wind, and animals.

At 1.9 miles, you will plunge back into the woods once again just before the path joins the nature trail at the yellow post. Turn left here and follow the nature trail back to the trailhead and the parking lot.

■ MORE FUN

The Discovery Center natural history museum has excellent displays. Located near the dog fields and picnic area at the far end of the parking lot, it is open Saturdays between Memorial Day and Labor Day, and admission is free.

■ TO THE TRAILHEAD

Starting out from the intersection with Capital City Freeway, on CA 99 drive 32 miles south to Lodi. Leave the highway at West Turner Road, Exit 267a. Turn left on West Turner and drive 1.7 miles to the park entrance on the right, on Laurel Avenue (directly opposite Superburger Drive-In). Drive down the lane and turn right when the large oak in the road causes you to slow down, and park inside the gate. The trailhead is directly adjacent to the lot.

■ OVERVIEW

LENGTH: 3 miles	**MAPS:** USGS Ripon; local map at entry kiosk
CONFIGURATION: Loop	
WATER REQUIRED: 1 liter	**WHEELCHAIR TRAVERSABLE:** Access on Grey Fox and part of River Bend Trail
SCENERY: Riparian forest	
EXPOSURE: Shaded trail	**FACILITIES:** Trailhead toilets and water; picnic tables; camping
TRAFFIC: Light	
TRAIL SURFACE: Duff and dirt	**DRIVING DISTANCE:** 63.5 miles
HIKING TIME: 1.5 hours	**SPECIAL COMMENTS:** This is a great trail for children on a hot day. The trail is wide, shaded, and surrounded by wonderful plants and animals.
SEASON: Year-round, 8 a.m.–sunset	
ACCESS: $6 fee	

■ SNAPSHOT

These easy trails loop through the magnificent valley oaks and towering cottonwoods of this rare riparian forest. A hike through this forest draped with wild grapevines and filled with the song of various birds will be remembered even by children for a long time. Excellent interpretive signage also makes this hike an educational trip for adults as well as children.

■ CLOSE-UP

Only about 5 percent of California's original Central Valley riparian forest remains. Located on the Stanislaus River, the Caswell Memorial State Park (MSP) has preserved an impressive expanse of woodland, 258 acres of this rare California ecosystem that once stretched for miles toward the mountains.

If you begin at the restrooms, your trailhead is at the end of the walkway leading west past the picnic tables and the seating area. An informational kiosk at the trailhead displays a

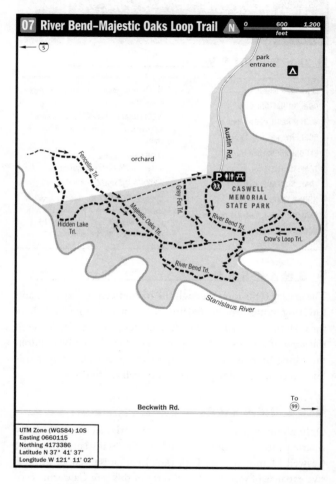

UTM Zone (WGS84) 10S
Easting 0660115
Northing 4173386
Latitude N 37° 41' 37"
Longitude W 121° 11' 02"

general map of the park, along with descriptions of the flora and fauna one might encounter in this park.

Hikers in wheelchairs can access the first 0.25 miles of the River Bend Trail. Connect to the Grey Fox Trail for a 0.7-mile loop. These trails are made of smooth, packed dirt, so those in wheelchairs may need some assistance along both the trails.

Past the signs for the trailhead, towering valley oaks and cottonwoods cast shade across the trail, and any light that might sneak in is caught by the curtain of wild grapevines draped from the trees. Immediately after they are made, the sounds of owls calling and woodpeckers hammering are muffled. Your footsteps are almost silent as you proceed along this dirt-and-duff trail on the way to the next interpretive sign.

Rather than just listing the species of this riparian habitat, the signs in Caswell MSP relate a natural scenario in terms that are easy for children to remember. You will pass an area close to the river, where a sign cautions hikers to stay back from the eroding bank. After that, the trail is wide and there is minimal poison oak.

Head into the Crow's Loop Trail by taking the next two left turns. Blackberries and sedges both thrive in this flood-plain, growing amid the poison oak. There are some nice vistas of the river here as long as you stay on the trail. Although it is not as manicured as the interpretive section, this 0.4-mile loop gives one some insight into the variety of this ecosystem's wildlife. Raccoons, foxes, skunks, weasels, and squirrels have all left evidence of their passing. Most of the smaller mammals, such as the riparian brush rabbit and the riparian wood rat, take up residence in the thick understory and rarely venture farther than 50 feet from their burrow or nest. And for good reason. Sitting at the bottom of the food chain, they are meals for raptors such as great horned owls, osprey, and Swainson's hawks; they are also on the menu of all the mammals listed above; they are even taken by snakes. No wonder they live in seclusion.

When you are halfway around the loop, the branches of valley oaks will fill the sky above your trail and block the horizon. Pass through a grove of young sycamores to finish this loop. Take the same two left forks you passed previously to return to the River Bend Trail. Every intersection in this park is marked with a brown wooden post signed with trail names and directional arrows, so you should have no worries about becoming disoriented in this thickly forested park.

In about 100 feet, you will stay on River Bend Trail by turning left at the intersection with the Grey Fox Trail. Follow the River Bend Trail with the river on your left as you head south. As you walk in and out of the shade, your path is interrupted by a horizontal oak that offers no options other than scrambling through its broken limbs and over its trunk as the blackberries on the other side beckon and the wild rose perfumes the air. The poison oak reminds you to watch what you grab.

There are plenty of side trails to the edge of the Stanislaus River. Here you can watch for the occasional turtle as it suns itself on a stick poking out of the mud bank. The trail remains a wide doubletrack despite the overgrowth of sedges. More frequently now, cottonwoods tower 75 feet over your track. The trail is totally shaded for the next five to ten minutes on even the sunniest day. Look down for a bit to spot the next two turns. Take a left at the intersection that puts you on Majestic Oaks Trail. (Straight ahead would take you to the parking lot.) Walk just 100 feet and take another left back onto River Bend Trail.

Geese can often be heard arguing on the river as you walk through the wild grapevines, but you'll be unable to see past the greenery to the water. Continue to the junction with Hidden Lake Trail. Make a left on this trail, heading southwest. (From this point, you can reach the Fenceline Trail by walking 50 feet ahead.) As you walk along Hidden Lake Trail (it could have been called the Active Raccoon Trail for the plentiful markings of these nocturnal mammals), you will encounter another fallen oak where a trail enters from the right. Signed as the Mosquito Trail, it does not appear on the park map. Our route goes forward in search of Hidden Lake.

Perhaps there is a lake hidden in the thick forest that this trail skirts, but light does not penetrate far enough to reveal any sort of secret fishing spot here. Regardless, the trail is soft, the shade is cool, and the wild rose is relaxing. Notice that some small areas of the forest have been thinned by burning; the Yokut people did the same thing when they lived in this area. Look for green or brown narrow fiber tubes standing in these thinned areas: they protect valley oak seedlings as they gain a foothold in the forest. Hike onward to a right turn at Fenceline Trail, where Rabbit's Run Trail leads off to the left, then hike along Fenceline Trail about 0.25 miles. The duff-covered road is bordered by the orchard to your left and valley oaks to your right. You can see many more of the seedling tubes here as you approach a junction with River Bend Trail. Continue on to your left and pass a wood-chipping area. In a moment, you will take a right onto Majestic Oaks Trail. Aside from the huge valley oaks with their spreading canopies, there are numerous seedlings planted and protected here for future generations to enjoy.

Pass the next two intersections; they are both part of the River Bend Trail. Take in the vast numbers of valley oaks that grow here. They are magnificent and will be here for a while, thanks to the care of this park and the Caswell family.

Turn north on Gray Fox Trail, where the interpretive signage continues. Blackberries and roses on one side and grapes overhead bound your trail an hour into the hike. When you reach the fence line, turn right toward the parking lot. The corner of the orchard is to your left, and the trail enters the parking lot at the northwest corner.

■ TO THE TRAILHEAD

From the intersection of the Capital City Freeway and CA 99 South, drive 58 miles south toward Stockton on CA 99. Just past CA 120, exit at Austin Road, cross the railroad tracks, and drive south 5.1 miles on Austin Road, cruising through orchards to reach the Caswell Memorial State Park entrance. The entry kiosk is 100 feet ahead. After paying your entry fee and picking up a map, drive 0.4 miles to the end of the shaded road. Turn left into the parking lot. Restrooms are at the east end of the lot, and the trailhead is toward the west end, near the information kiosk.

08 Grizzly Island Wildlife Area Trail

■ OVERVIEW

LENGTH: 4.5 miles

CONFIGURATION: Balloon

WATER REQUIRED: 1 liter

SCENERY: Delta marshland

EXPOSURE: Fully exposed to sun and wind. Ear protection, hat, windbreaker, and gloves may be needed any time of year. The temperature here will be several degrees lower than in the valley.

TRAFFIC: Minimal

TRAIL SURFACE: Dirt and grass

HIKING TIME: 2 hours

SEASON: Feb.–July, sunrise–sunset

ACCESS: $2.50 admission; free with one of several state permits. Open for hunting seasons; call ahead for hiking dates. Check with Dept. of Fish and Game for closures and permit details.

MAPS: USGS Honker Bay; area map in office or at www.dfg.ca.gov/lands/wa/region3/grizzlyisland.html

FACILITIES: Pit toilet at trailhead

WHEELCHAIR TRAVERSABLE: No

DRIVING DISTANCE: 57 miles

SPECIAL COMMENTS: This is an unsigned route on levee roads. Levee roads may lead to dead ends or small adventures. Do not leave the levee roads, even for short distances.

■ SNAPSHOT

Carved out of the Suisun Marsh, the largest contiguous saltwater marsh on the West Coast, the Grizzly Island Wildlife Area offers an abundance of wildlife and botanical diversity. This short hike lets hikers walk slowly enough to quietly observe amphibians, reptiles, and fish; waterfowl, songbirds, and raptors; and burrowing mammals, grazing mammals, and predatory mammals. At any given moment along this trail, the alert hiker will be able to spot easily identified specimens, whether it's turtles, frogs, otters, or skunks. .

■ CLOSE-UP

The informative kiosks at the Department of Fish and Game (DFG) Field Office provide a good overview. Inside the office there are more displays that hint at the diversity of wildlife here.

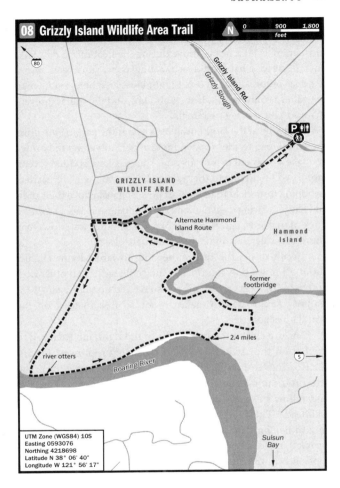

08 Grizzly Island Wildlife Area Trail

N   0   900   1,800
feet

80

Grizzly Island Rd.

Grizzly Slough

P

GRIZZLY ISLAND
WILDLIFE AREA

Alternate Hammond
Island Route

Hammond
Island

former
footbridge

2.4 miles

5

river otters

Roaring River

Suisun
Bay

UTM Zone (WGS84) 10S
Easting 0593076
Northing 4218698
Latitude N 38° 06' 40"
Longitude W 121° 56' 17"

The Suisin Marsh Natural History Association Web site, **www
.suisunwildlife.org,** includes lists of species found on Grizzly
Island that you can use for quick reference. Such lists make it
easy to recall all you have viewed.

Binoculars will help the patient hiker spot a surprising number of species. Morning and late afternoon are best because most animals tend not to move during the heat of the day. Hikers will need a hat with a brim, sunglasses, sunscreen, and a wind jacket or soft-shell top. Light gloves also help, even when the valley is quite warm. Insects abound, and the trail is uneven, thanks to burrowing mammals.

Starting at the large eucalyptus tree at the parking lot, cross the gravel road to the wooden footbridge. Stop along the bridge and take a moment to look around. You may have spotted several raptors while driving to the trailhead. Here you will see harriers swooping from field to field, kites hovering just above their prey, and hawks soaring even higher. For no apparent reason, an entire flock of mallards, egrets, or any of a dozen other waterfowl may churn the water and air to get somewhere else fast.

Walk across the bridge, heading toward Mount Diablo, about 15 miles due south from the trailhead eucalyptus. Legend holds that Grizzly Island was so named because bears from Mount Diablo used to make an annual trek to feast on the island's blackberries.

At the end of the bridge, zig to the right and then zag to the left on the obvious levee road, heading southwest toward the Roaring River. At 0.6 miles, a levee road will enter from the left. (You can take an alternate route from this point. Turn left and follow this road, taking two left turns to get back to the trailhead.) This hike continues 0.2 miles farther down the trail to another junction. Your choices are to cross the canal and turn left, make a U-turn to the left, or turn left over the culvert pipe and continue on the dirt tracks.

The hike described here turns left over the pipe and heads slightly southwest on the dirt tracks. Mount Diablo, off to the southeast, can act as your guide. More directly east are the large wind turbines that harness the constant gusts to busily churn out electricity. It is common to spot tule elk in the highlands around the island. They were successfully reintroduced to the marshes in the late 1970s.

Along this short stretch of dirt trail, travel may be difficult in wet weather. Take the next left in 0.7 miles, noticing the steep edges of the slough. In midday none were active, but river otters left their marks here. Tracks and signs of other mammals were also frozen in the muddy margins of the sloughs and shallow ditches. Sometimes our own senses provide us all the clues we need to identify a mammal. Very close encounters with very active skunks are a real possibility. Let your nose be your guide in turning away whenever the odor intensifies. These trails are choked with tall grasses and weeds or have grass-constricted margins that can conceal any manner of creatures. Keep a sharp lookout for a T-intersection just before you walk into the slough.

Another left turn and another 0.7 miles—to the east this time. Your left-turn marker is the point at which you are directly south of the trailhead eucalyptus. So far you have traveled 2.4 miles. It is just a short walk north to another T-intersection; take a right there. When a pheasant cock takes flight as you approach, try to stay on the trail and in your boots. They go from 0 to 60 miles per hour right underfoot.

Navigation is easy, and you can see your trailhead, so spend some time crawling along the margins of the slough, where the amphibians and reptiles spend their days. Western pond turtles enjoy warming in the sun along a log or on a muddy bank. The two-tone green Pacific tree frog may surprise you with its voice but if you are sharp enough to spot one, you will see that its call far outweighs its body size.

Turn left at the next intersection and then make another left before you run into the water at the dilapidated footbridge. You will now be heading generally northwest. Your winding trail parallels the trail along the opposite shore of Hammond Island. (That is the alternate trail that was mentioned above.)

Your next intersection is a repeat of your confusing first turn. Cross over the culvert and turn right, toward your trail-head tree. If you prefer a longer hike from this point, in just 0.2 miles you can turn right to follow the margins of Hammond Island, circumnavigating it back to the trailhead parking lot.

Just turn left twice and you will be back at the trailhead with more stories.

The great thing about Grizzly Island is its concentration of wildlife and its network of levee roads, all of which are open to hikers. And, remember, dead ends are just a reason to enjoy your trail twice.

■ MORE FUN

Nearby Rush Ranch is a 2,070-acre open space that protects important brackish tidal marshes. For details on its many offerings, including hiking, see its Web site, **www.rushranch.org.**

The Delta region has several preserves and parks with interpretive nature trails. The Cosumnes River Preserve (Hike 5) and Caswell Memorial State Park both have excellent interpretive trails.

■ TO THE TRAILHEAD

Drive 38 miles west on Interstate 80 to CA 12 East (Exit 43) in Suisun City. Follow CA 12, Rio Vista Road, 3.8 miles to Grizzly Island Road, where you will turn south. This turn is directly across from the shopping center at Sunset Avenue. As you drive south around the Potrero Hills, you may notice an immediate change of scenery from valley to delta. About 5.5 miles from your turn south onto Grizzly Island Road, you will make a right turn across the bridge and boat-launch ramps at Montezuma Slough; the transition is unmistakable. Another 3.5 miles and you will be greeted by signs requesting you register at the DFG office. After registering and looking at the displays inside, continue 5.6 miles straight ahead on the gravel-and-dirt road (bear left whenever given a choice) until you see the towering eucalyptus tree at the signed parking lot 3. There is plenty of parking here and a portable toilet but no water.

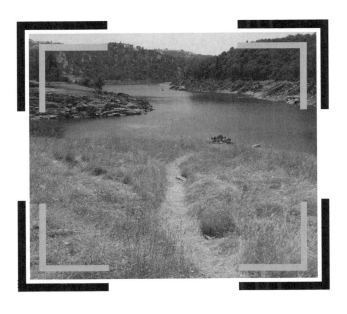

Foothills Hikes

■ OVERVIEW

LENGTH: 1.8 miles	**ACCESS:** $6 day-use fee
CONFIGURATION: Connected loops	**MAPS:** USGS Pine Grove; local map in park brochure
WATER REQUIRED: 1 liter	
SCENERY: Foothill woodland and grassland	**WHEELCHAIR TRAVERSABLE:** Partly, near grinding rocks and other exhibits
EXPOSURE: Shady, except at midday	**FACILITIES:** Restrooms, water, camping
TRAFFIC: Moderate	**DRIVING DISTANCE:** 55 miles
TRAIL SURFACE: Dirt and duff, asphalt	**SPECIAL COMMENTS:** The Indian Grinding Rock has the most mortar holes of any grinding rock in North America.
HIKING TIME: 1 hour	
SEASON: Year-round, sunrise–sunset	

■ SNAPSHOT

The trails around the 135-acre Indian Grinding Rock State Historic Park pass exhibits, plants, reconstructions—including a Miwok village and a ceremonial round house—and the famous Indian Grinding Rock, Chaw'se. Having nearly 1,200 mortars on its bedrock limestone, this is the largest number of bedrock mortars anywhere in North America. Still visible next to some of the mortars are 2,000-to-3,000-year-old petroglyphs.

■ CLOSE-UP

The two trails—the North Trail and the South Nature Trail—can be joined conveniently to create a loop that encompasses all of the park's sights. There is no route-finding necessary because all the trails are well marked and easily identified. This loop starts at the trailhead in front of the museum.

Head up the stone steps and walk along the trail as it trends northeast above the parking area. Walking between the road and the entrance drive, you will pass under incense cedars,

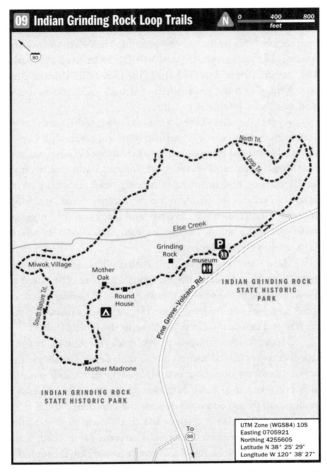

09 Indian Grinding Rock Loop Trails

N

0   400   800
feet

80

North Trl.

Loop Trl.

Else Creek

Grinding
Rock

P

museum

Miwok Village

Mother
Oak

Round
House

South Nature Trl.

Pine Grove–Volcano Rd.

INDIAN GRINDING ROCK
STATE HISTORIC
PARK

Mother Madrone

INDIAN GRINDING ROCK
STATE HISTORIC PARK

To
88

UTM Zone (WGS84) 10S
Easting 0705921
Northing 4255605
Latitude N 38° 25' 29"
Longitude W 120° 38' 27"

foothill pines, and live oaks. Some faint-purple brodiaeas add color to the trailside. A footbridge keeps your feet dry as you cross the head of Else Creek, named for one of the area's original farming families. Look ahead for the hole in the wooden fence, where you will cross the road.

The farmhouse to your right was an original pioneer homestead. In the late 1880s, the land here was sold to Serafino Scapuccino, who protected the grinding-rock area and whose family sold the farm to the state in 1958 to be used as a park. The orchards here provided fruits for miners in Volcano and elsewhere. Continue your northward walk under some huge madrone and whiteleaf manzanita.

A junction offers hikers a choice between the lower Loop Trail or the upper North Trail. Both trails feature foothill woodland and grassland ecosystems. Small clearings between manzanita display colorful irises and lupines, and buttercups, monkeyflower, and brodiaea border the trail. Towering overhead are Douglas fir, ponderosa pine, incense cedar, and foothill pine, all mixed in with live oak and black oak. But none of these specimens shines like the majestic valley oak—of which there are huge examples here.

Head slightly uphill on the North Trail, a packed-dirt path that winds in and out of the madrone and pine. The scent of needles baking in the sun fills the air. A grove of live oak provides some cool shade at midday, when the sun breaks through onto the trail just before the Loop Trail rejoins the North Trail.

Meander down some easy switchbacks through the manzanita on this rock-lined section of the trail. Fence lizards are the only critters scurrying about in the heat of the day, and they reveal their every step in the dry duff littering the forest floor. Cross a small runoff stream and head down some improvised steps.

Your trail takes a distinct left turn downhill toward the first valley oaks to come into view. Cross the gravel road, making a slight jog to your right, and continue walking through the tall grass bordering a much narrower trail. A sign displays the distance to junctions and park features.

Ahead of you on the right is a grove of valley oaks in which all of the oaks are more than 300 years old. With the support of their enormous trunks, these trees spread majestically across the meadow, creating a shaded parklike setting. A small footbridge helps hikers across Else Creek at the end of the meadow. Incense cedars and native grasses lead hikers up to the Miwok village reconstruction at the junction with the South Nature Trail.

The Miwok settled a broad area between the Cosumnes River to the north and the Calaveras River to the south. Because acorns were a staple food crop, the Miwok were attracted to this area, which has groves of valley oaks and a broad, flat rock on which to grind the nuts into flour. One wonders if the trees were here before the rock was discovered, or if their proliferation was a result of the grinding rock's use.

After inspecting the round cedar-bark houses in the village, turn right onto the South Nature Trail and start looking for interpretive-marker posts—about three feet tall, brown, numbered, and hard to spot. The interpretive guide for sale in the museum will steer you.

Towering incense cedar, Douglas fir, ponderosa pine, sugar pine, and valley oak shade your downhill trail as you cross a creek and enter a rather open area right up against fenced-in private property. Blackberry, iris, and columbine grow in this moist, cool area, along with ferns and kit-kit-dizze, which crowd the trailside.

Winding around a bit brings you to a spectacularly large madrone. Fire-scarred and weather-beaten, it is surrounded by iris and lupine. The trail continues north past a trailside bench.

The trail borders the campgrounds to their left and passes a grand incense cedar with an imposing split trunk that reaches eight feet in diameter. Trail markers will keep you on track when you are about to walk into the picnic tables. Jog slightly left and stay close to the fence around the campsites. Watch for signs directing hikers to the park's features. The grandest living feature of the park is the Mother Oak—a 600-year-old valley oak that spreads across the meadow. It is an awesome natural wonder and an imposing presence not found in most parks.

Valley oaks also shade the entrance to the ceremonial

Round House, which is one of the largest in California. Continue along the walk to the grinding rock itself. The grinding rock is a bedrock formation of marbleized limestone. Having 1,185 individual grinding holes, it is the largest such collection of mortars in North America. The rock's use has been dated to 2,000 to 3,000 years ago. Beside some of the mortars are petroglyphs—pictorial representations carved in the stone— which show important everyday objects such as nets, the sun, and man himself. A viewing platform allows for close-up views of the entire rock.

   Return to the museum trailhead by walking past the bark houses and the metal sculpture of a Miwok Indian dancer.

■ MORE FUN

The Chaw'se Indian Museum next to the trailhead has excellent Miwok displays and natural history exhibits, and is particularly oriented to children, with many hands-on displays.

■ TO THE TRAILHEAD

From downtown Sacramento, drive 3 miles east on US 50 to the Howe Avenue exit toward Rancho Murieta. Drive southeast 18 miles on the Jackson Road to Rancho Murieta, then about 13.5 miles to the CA 49 junction (the second right turn); drive 7 miles south to Sutter Creek and another 4 miles to Jackson. Turn left on CA 88 and drive 8 miles to Pine Grove. Turn-left onto Pine Grove–Volcano Road toward Volcano. In about 1 mile, a sign on the left indicates the campground. The park entrance is 0.25 miles past this on the left. The trailhead, marked by a directional arrow, is at the end of the sidewalk that leads into the museum.

■ OVERVIEW

LENGTH: 4.1 miles	**ACCESS:** $7 parking fee
CONFIGURATION: Out-and-back	**MAPS:** USGS Pilot Hill
WATER REQUIRED: 1 liter	**FACILITIES:** Gravel parking area; picnic tables and pit toilets at boat ramp
SCENERY: Foothill forest surrounding lake	
	WHEELCHAIR TRAVERSABLE: No
EXPOSURE: Shaded, with patches of sun	**DRIVING DISTANCE:** 21.3 miles
TRAFFIC: Moderate	**SPECIAL COMMENTS:** Historic North Fork Ditch parallels trail. The Pioneer Express Trail crosses the main road and continues from Rattlesnake Bar to Horseshoe Bar.
TRAIL SURFACE: Dirt and duff	
HIKING TIME: 2 hours	
SEASON: Year-round, sunrise–sunset	

■ SNAPSHOT

The hike to Avery's Pond is a great adventure for children and parents who want a brief yet interesting hike. This route takes you past Avery's Pond and the Newcastle powerhouse at Mormon's Ravine. The trail guides hikers along remnants of the North Fork Ditch, which supplied water to mining camps and towns along the American River.

■ CLOSE-UP

After gold was discovered in the South Fork of the American River in 1848, mining camps sprang up along both the South Fork and the North Fork. Men from every corner of the world worked this river: England, Scotland, Wales, New York, Virginia, Kentucky, New South Wales, Hawaii, and China. They stayed with their claims, camping right beside their river workplace. The camps turned into towns and, no matter the size, each settlement was given a name—colorful, descriptive names such as Rattlesnake Bar, Mormon Bar, Mormon Ravine, Oregon Bar,

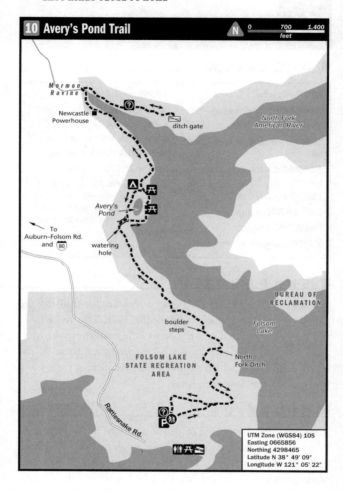

10 Avery's Pond Trail

N   0   700   1,400
                  feet

Mormon Ravine

Newcastle Powerhouse

ditch gate

North Fork American River

Avery's Pond

watering hole

To Auburn–Folsom Rd. and 80

BUREAU OF RECLAMATION

Folsom Lake

boulder steps

North Fork Ditch

FOLSOM LAKE STATE RECREATION AREA

Rattlesnake Rd.

UTM Zone (WGS84) 10S
Easting 0665856
Northing 4298465
Latitude N 38° 49' 09"
Longitude W 121° 05' 22"

and Manhattan Bar. Some establishments disappeared overnight, but others persisted. In 1865 Rattlesnake Bar was a town of more than 1,000 residents. Avery's Pond and some sights along the way are relics from the gold-mining days along the North Fork of the American River.

Leave the horse-assembly area at the signed trailhead at the northeast end of the parking lot. Your trail starts out as a dirt path that becomes a doubletrack in short order. When the wide track veers right, stay on the single path that leads left. The doubletrack will rejoin your path shortly. The meadow you are crossing is filled with wildflowers in the spring. A sign ahead proclaims that you are on the Pioneer Express Trail and indicates the distance to Avery's Pond and Auburn.

After you head generally east for about ten minutes, the trail turns north to meander through live oak and toyon. After 0.25 miles, you will start descending a bit along a deeply rutted section of trail. As you reach a sunny hillside, look to the opposite shore of the lake where the "bathtub rings" in the dirt bespeak the various lake levels over the years. Just as you near 0.5 miles, with the lake in full view, you may be distracted by a turkey or two as they flash by looking very intent on their way to somewhere. Above, foothill pines shade the trail while the manzanita blazes with bright-red berries, which are sticky— like its flowers.

Walk along in the cool shade of black oak, live oak, and more manzanita until you come to an easy but steep downhill stretch. A large outcrop to your left leans out over the trail. Well protected by poison oak, these rocks are not the type one would be enthusiastic about bouldering. The trail is crossed with smaller boulders that serve as stairs to help you clamber down the trail. Your path is now sand and pea gravel and travels alongside the lake about 50 feet above the shoreline. The trail runs up next to a steep drop to the rocks below just as you see the first signs of the North Fork Ditch. Here you can see views of the lake as it disappears into the foothills.

Cross a small drainage ditch just before you come upon a large patch of blackberries at about the 1-mile point. The ditch is plainly visible for the next mile. Encrusted with blackberries, the ditch runs to your right. Below you is another section of the concrete wall that comprised part of the ditch. Moisture-loving blackberries are the main plant here, offering themselves to hikers at many points along the trail.

Under a nice cover of shade is a horse-watering trough fed by the spring just on the other side of the bridge at the pond. The wooden bridge crossing the aqueduct was restored in 1994 in an Eagle Scout project. Walk another 175 feet to cross another bridge, which signals your arrival at the pond. Turn right and head toward the lake. Look to the right of the trail and you will see Sierra iris growing among the live oak.

You will find a picnic table about halfway around the pond, next to a lonely live oak tree surrounded by scant vegetation. This spot is totally exposed and might not be the best for a picnic, but the trails that lead to both the lake and the pond indicate that this could be a good fishing spot. Be careful: the bank surrounding the pond is steep, and the pond is not suitable for swimming or wading.

For excellent shade while you picnic, there are tables located farther along the pond trail just before the next junction on the left, and also just after it on the right. If you want to circumnavigate the pond, continue left at the next junction and make your way along the north shore of the pond. There is a bit more to see in the vicinity.

About 0.5 miles ahead is a small hydroelectric plant operated by PG&E. To get there, take the right-hand trail at the junction and you will walk roughly parallel to the road you see above you to the left. You will reach the road in a matter of seconds. Take notice of the mountain lion warning posted on the tree. Follow the road down as it turns to gravel, and then around the bend; you will see the small hydro facility—the Newcastle power plant—ahead. It was built in 1986 and produces electricity for up to 12,000 homes.

As you walk toward the power plant, you can see the point at which the North Fork enters the lake. The powerful stream creates a wide ravine here and drops a jumble of rocks and debris in its wake. Look closely and you will probably see deer feeding amid the willows and sedges growing in this tributary. The South Fork's entrance to the lake near Salmon Falls is 5.5 miles directly southeast of your current position; you can imagine the commerce that occurred between miners on both rivers. According to historical accounts, a bridge was built in 1862 at Rattlesnake Bar that served for almost 100 years, until a truck full of "fertilizer" sparked the bridge's collapse in 1954.

Pass the modern plant now, and follow the trail across another bridge at Mormon Ravine just past the power plant. Turn right and continue through the wooded area above the river. Look below you on the right, and you can plainly see sections of the water ditch. Follow the trail until, at the 2-mile point, you come to an informational kiosk that highlights the hydro facility and provides some brief history regarding your trail.

The large, open field above you to the left fills with wildflowers each spring. Wally baskets, brodiaea, buttercups, and blue dicks sprinkle the hillside with color. Startle a deer from its afternoon slumber here and see who jumps higher. (Answer: the deer. Repeatedly. But nice try anyway.) This trail continues to Auburn, where it begins above the Auburn Dam site. As you look right to the live oak about ten feet off the trail, you may notice a concrete structure. A little investigation uncovers what appears to be a ditch gate, long since disused.

This is a convenient spot to turn around. You have hiked 2 miles, and your small hiking companions are surely ready for refreshments back at the trailhead. Retrace your steps until you come to the pond, and take the right-hand fork at the junction. Walk through an environmental campsite with a few picnic tables. Just before you cross the bridge at the west end of the pond, look right to see more of the concrete sections of the ditch.

When you near the trailhead, you have a choice. Either retrace your steps exactly from the junction of the singletrack and the doubletrack, or take the fork to the right, startle some more turkeys in the woods, and then emerge at the kiosk adjacent to the trailhead.

■ TO THE TRAILHEAD

From the intersection with Capital City Freeway, drive 15 miles east on Interstate 80 to Loomis, and exit at Horseshoe Bar Road. Turn left at the end of the ramp onto Horseshoe Bar Road; bear left and then take the next left turn onto Horseshoe Bar Road. Continue 3.4 miles to Auburn–Folsom Road. Turn left and drive 2.3 miles to Newcastle Road, where you will turn right and go 1 mile to Rattlesnake Road. Turn right again and follow the road another mile until the pavement ends. Stop and self-register at the entry kiosk. Drive 0.2 miles to the sign for the horse-assembly area and boat launch. Turn left and drive 0.4 miles to the sign for the horse-assembly area, then turn left again, into the gravel parking lot. The signed trailhead is at the northeast end of the lot, in the grass.

■ OVERVIEW

LENGTH: 5.1 miles	**MAPS:** USGS Gold Hill. An excellent color map of all the trails is available online at www.placer.ca.gov/Departments/Facility/parks/hiddenfalls.aspx.
CONFIGURATION: Connected loops	
WATER REQUIRED: 2 liters	
SCENERY: Riparian and foothill woodland	**FACILITIES:** Restrooms, water fountain, and pay telephone
EXPOSURE: Well-shaded trail most of the way	**WHEELCHAIR TRAVERSABLE:** Yes. The Hidden Gateway Trail is accessible and begins just 10 feet past the trailhead for this hike.
TRAFFIC: Very little	
TRAIL SURFACE: Sand and rock; dirt and duff	
HIKING TIME: 2–3 hours	**DRIVING DISTANCE:** 32 miles
SEASON: Year-round, sunrise–sunset	**SPECIAL COMMENTS:** Scenic, new trail system on 220 acres being expanded to 1,180 acres
ACCESS: No fees or permits	

■ SNAPSHOT

Hidden Falls Regional Park, a new addition in Placer County's Placer Legacy Program, is a model for suburban open-space design and use. The park's 7 miles of trails are available to hikers, bikers, runners, and horseback riders. An accessible trail—the Hidden Gateway Trail—offers excellent views of the 220-acre site. The other paths consist of either loops or out-and-back trails that range from moderate to difficult. The hike described here combines portions of each trail to give the hiker a solid workout rewarded by excellent scenery. These trails are well marked, and intersections are somewhat frequent, so being temporarily disoriented should not be a concern on this hike.

■ CLOSE-UP

Your trail, which starts out near the top of the ridge, descends to Deadman's Creek and then ascends the next ridge to the

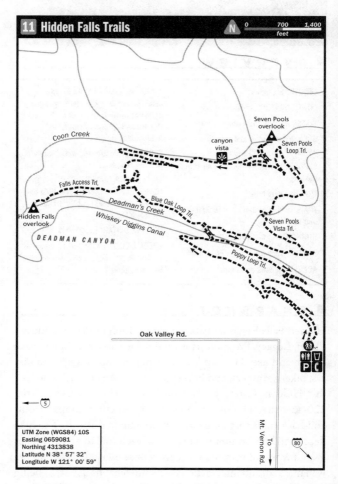

11 Hidden Falls Trails

N   0   700   1,400
              feet

Coon Creek

Seven Pools overlook

canyon vista

Seven Pools Loop Trl.

Falls Access Trl.

Blue Oak Loop Trl.

Deadman's Creek

Hidden Falls overlook

Whiskey Diggins Canal

Seven Pools Vista Trl.

DEADMAN CANYON

Poppy Loop Trl.

Oak Valley Rd.

5

Mt. Vernon Rd.

To
80

UTM Zone (WGS84) 10S
Easting 0659081
Northing 4313838
Latitude N 38° 57' 32"
Longitude W 121° 00' 59"

north before arriving at the pools of Coon Creek. The nicely shaded path takes you along Coon Creek as you make your way west toward Deadman's Falls.

Your trail starts at the information kiosk at the end of the parking lot, where you will see a map of the complete trail system. The restrooms and pay phone are to your left; walk about five feet down the sidewalk, turn right, and descend a few concrete steps to the dirt path of Poppy Loop Trail, and then turn left and begin walking north.

As you start down Poppy Loop Trail, the view to your east is of fenced cattle ranches ringed by foothill woodland forests. This old four-wheel-drive road is rather exposed as you descend to the first U-turn. The trail you see to the right is your return route.

On the way down, though, you will feel a significant cooling as you enter the shade of live oak and foothill pine. Within moments you will begin to hear Deadman's Creek. Another, more appetizing, sign of the upcoming creek is the appearance of miner's lettuce on the left side of your trail. Resist the temptation to pick—it is prohibited—as you head toward the bridge ahead of you.

Crossing the bridge, you are on Pond Turtle Trail. Take this connector 30 feet to the junction with Blue Oak Loop Trail. A sharp right uphill puts you on the side of the hill under the shade of the foothill woodland understory—toyon and manzanita. This trail will quickly gain elevation and then level off. To your left you can see the contours of the hills in the trail cut. Notice the gentle folds of the rock strata as you pass.

After you round a seasonal runoff ravine from the left, you may begin to notice more blue oak—much of it speckled with oakmoss lichen. On the right, a rather large—and horizontal—foothill pine stretches from its roots at the canyon center to its crown tip at the trailside. Signs indicate this tree fell during the winter of 2006. Your trail continues to gain elevation after it swings back to the north. Walking in the shade, watch for weasel signs, which are usually plumb in the middle of the trail.

As you level out after 1.4 miles, you will see a signpost (labeled #10) at the junction where you now leave the Blue Oak Loop when it turns left and you continue straight onto the Seven Pools Vista Trail.

Descend a bit to the northeast toward the Seven Pools area. You will not actually reach the pools on this trail. It is the next junction that will get you there. For now, the dirt- and leaf-covered trail seems like the easy part of the hike: gently descending, continuously shaded, quiet enough to hear birds and the stream.

Among the toyon, manzanita, and live oak, the trail will make a U-turn before reaching the Seven Pools area and will then wrap around the hillside, gently descending in and out of a ravine before reaching a well-signed intersection with Seven Pools Loop. Your route turns sharply right, onto Seven Pools Loop, at signpost #11.

Head east, descending just below the previous trail section, getting ever closer to Coon Creek. To help keep your feet dry, use the small bridge that crosses the ravine you walked around earlier. Now head north about 100 yards to a spur trail that leads to a rock outcrop looking over the cascades and into one of the pools.

Return to the Seven Pools Loop, heading west. Notice the bits and chunks of quartz rock along this section of trail. Quartz-bearing gravels attracted miners' attention, as the mining ditch along Deadman's Creek reminds us. The large blocks in the creek bottom testify to the general geological makeup of this region: highly fractured blocks and faults, squeezed, uplifted, folded, coated with lava and mudflows, washed, scrubbed, bleached, and left as you find them today. To see a good example, just before reaching the vista ahead on the right, look at the outcrop of rock running from the left on the hill above you. It continues immediately under your feet, and out to your right at the boulder-littered canyon floor.

Shortly after the vista spot, just as the trail turns away from the creek, your path crosses Pond Turtle Trail. This junction is simple: keep walking straight. But if you want a pleasant spot to sit for a moment, the creek is right there.

Continuing west on Seven Pools Loop, the trail varies from 5 to 50 feet above the creek bed. Walk past any blocked trails that are marked for trail restoration. The 960-acre ranch to the west is currently being surveyed for additional trails, but requires vegetation recovery in some areas first.

The Seven Pools Loop will switchback, ascending to the east for 0.2 miles. Turning right at the intersection with Quail Run Trail will send you toward the Falls Access Trail for one of the real highlights of this hike.

As you round the curve of Quail Run Trail, resist the temptation to shortcut the ten feet across to the Falls Access Trail. Restoration of that impromptu trail is in progress and needs cooperation.

Walk another 150 feet around the curve. Just after the contorted black and burgundy madrone, take a right at the junction onto Blue Oak Loop. Walk 75 feet, then turn right onto the Falls Access Trail, heading west.

This is the most difficult section of the route. No horses or bikes are permitted on this trail for good reasons. The Falls Access Trail is the most uneven, least well-established trail in the park. It most closely approximates a typical wilderness use-trail. You will have some rocks and boulders to contend with, and the side trails are obvious enough to avoid. Descending to within 50 feet of Deadman's Creek, you will find compelling vista points overlooking some little riffles.

More importantly, this trail ends rather precipitously at the falls overlook, and the footing is quite slippery, so do not rush around that last bend! At least 100 feet before the trail's end, the falls and the viewpoint will be visible. Take a moment here to slow your pace. Before you drop down to the overlook, enjoy the view from this upper perch.

In March of 2007, Placer County engineers surveyed this spot to establish a platform overlook and picnic tables. A platform would be a distinct improvement because there is presently no way to see the entire falls without floating in midair. The 35-foot falls flow year-round. It is an impressive cataract that highlights the hike. Just below the falls is the junction with Coon Creek.

Return on this trail to the junction with the Blue Oak Loop, and turn right, heading southeast along the Blue Oak Loop. This section of the trail is flat and shaded. You are heading toward the bridge that ties the Blue Oak Loop with the Poppy Loop Trail.

When you cross the bridge on your return, turn left at the junction with the Poppy Loop Trail to walk along Deadman's Creek and past a massive blackberry patch. Three easy switchbacks lie between the creek and the ridge. Even though you leave the shade of foothill pines and California buckeyes for an open, dry slope, you cannot help but stop and admire the massive mistletoe-blotched valley oak that towers over the trail. Walk another 500 feet to the trailhead, with this giant to your right.

■ TO THE TRAILHEAD

From Interstate 80 East and Capitol City Freeway in Sacramento, drive 24 miles to Auburn. Exit CA 49 north toward Grass Valley. Drive north 2.7 miles; turn left onto Atwood Road, which becomes Mount Vernon Road after1.7 miles. Follow Mount Vernon Road 2.6 miles and turn right on Mears Drive. The Hidden Valley Regional Park entrance sign is up the hill on the right. Turn into the parking lot. The trailhead is to the right of the restrooms.

■ OVERVIEW

LENGTH: 4.4 miles	**MAPS:** USGS Auburn
CONFIGURATION: Out-and-back	**FACILITIES:** Pit toilet at North Fork Dam parking lot. Information kiosks and pit toilets are located about 150 feet south of the trailhead on the west side of Old Foresthill Road, and 200 feet west of the Old Foresthill Bridge on the north side of the road.
WATER REQUIRED: 1–2 liters, depending on season and time of day	
SCENERY: River views in a widening canyon lead up to a dammed lake	
EXPOSURE: Shaded trail, except during noon hours, in this north–south canyon	**WHEELCHAIR TRAVERSABLE:** No
TRAFFIC: Busy	**DRIVING DISTANCE:** 27.5 miles
TRAIL SURFACE: Sand, gravel, river rock, dirt, mud, and pavement	**SPECIAL COMMENTS:** This trail is also popular with mountain bikers. Most are courteous and will verbally "beep," but wise hikers will look over their shoulders frequently.
HIKING TIME: 2–3 hours	
SEASON: Year-round, sunrise–sunset	
ACCESS: No fees or permits	

■ SNAPSHOT

Lake Clementine Trail features the tallest bridge in California, gold-rush-era bridge remains, exposed Jurassic-period geology, riparian zone and foothill flora, a rock-lined swimming hole, and a tree-lined lake. A gentle grade offers some exercise along this 2.2-mile hike on a trail shared with runners and mountain bikers.

■ CLOSE-UP

The confluence of the North and Middle forks of the American River flows about 15 miles due north of the site where James Marshall first discovered gold on the South Fork of the American River. Since the time of the forty-niners, a dozen bridges have spanned these tributaries. Today four remain, three of which are used by motor vehicles. They are No Hands Bridge—

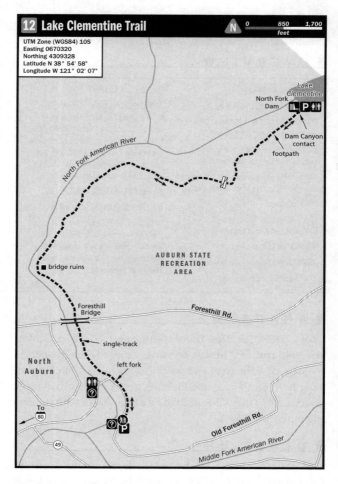

12 Lake Clementine Trail

UTM Zone (WGS84) 10S
Easting 0670320
Northing 4309328
Latitude N 38° 54' 58"
Longitude W 121° 02' 07"

N   0   850   1,700
feet

Lake Clementine

North Fork Dam

Dam Canyon contact footpath

North Fork American River

AUBURN STATE RECREATION AREA

bridge ruins

Foresthill Bridge

Foresthill Rd.

single-track

left fork

North Auburn

To 80

49

Old Foresthill Rd.

Middle Fork American River

formerly the Mountain Quarries RR Bridge and famous for its proximity to the finish of the Tevis Cup Trail Ride, the CA 49 bridge to Cool, Old Foresthill Road Bridge, and the most spectacular of all, Foresthill Bridge.

Lake Clementine Trail begins to the east of the confluence on the southeast side of Old Foresthill Road. The trailhead is marked by a gate signed TRAIL 139. Lined with boulders, this Jeep trail borders the east flank of the North Fork of the American River as it flows past you toward the confluence with the Middle Fork.

Your destination is at the end of a steady uphill amble to Lake Clementine, a lake created by the North Fork Dam, a debris dam built in 1939 by the Army Corps of Engineers. The flows along this fork of the American are not dam-controlled and so, as summer wanes, the waters below you become slower and warmer—making for great swimming opportunities. In late spring, by contrast, the high flow over the North Fork Dam creates spectacular mist and a thundering rumble.

Walking parallel to the river look left, to the west side, and you will see Stagecoach Trail, which climbs to join the route of an 1852 toll road known then as Yankee Jim's Turnpike. While you are looking, glance over your shoulder often because mountain bikers can approach quickly.

At about 1,000 feet from the trailhead, descend the first left fork toward the river's edge. A hundred feet farther, a stream crosses from your right. Take a moment to look left, though, to see the first of many bridge remains.

The biozones in this area—riparian and foothill woodland—are easy to tell apart because most of the riparian zone is on your left, and the river and the foothill woodland is on your right, along the canyon walls.

You'll see interior live oak, canyon live oak, madrone, foothill ("digger") pine, and California bay laurel. Watch for the spiky leaves of the toyon and the colorful redbuds interspersed with manzanita and poison oak.

As you look down the slope toward the river, you will pass cottonwoods, willows, valley oaks, and big-leaf maples. If the season is right, you'll also find an abundance of blackberries.

When the trail turns into a singletrack and hugs the river, you have walked a little more than half a mile. Bikers have no place to pass you here, so be alert. Look up and you will see the concrete pier and roadway of the Foresthill Bridge looming across the canyon. Walk about 500 feet and it will be directly overhead.

It's a record-setting 730 feet above the river, making it the tallest bridge in California and the third tallest in the United States. The bridge, built to carry traffic across the reservoir that would have been created by the Auburn Dam, was finished in 1973.

In the late 1970s, before the construction of the Auburn Dam, seismological risks were revealed and construction plans halted. Downriver from the confluence, a diversion tunnel was built that still stands. The dam's impact is most easily seen when you look up at the Foresthill Bridge: the water level would have reached just 22 feet below the top of the concrete pier above you.

After hiking 0.8 miles, look along both riverbanks for stone or concrete abutments marking original bridge sites. The concrete abutments were for the steel bridges of the early 20th century. Stone and rock abutments that supported several wooden bridges can be seen upriver within the next 0.3 miles.

Shaded by live oak and manzanita, boulder-lined pools of lazy, clear water lie within view. Stretching for almost a half mile, this portion of the river is known as Clark's Hole. Placer miners made dams of stacked boulders and river cobble, which formed these connected pools. The warm, slow waters here are now popular for swimming.

The midday sun at your back can be uncomfortable, and your moderately rolling trail has now turned into a fairly steady uphill exercise. To your right, the canyon wall rises sharply above you. The welcome coolness of ferns and mosses thriving wherever water seeps out of the manzanita-covered hillside helps relieve the heat.

The increasingly loud sound of water signals that you are approaching the North Fork Dam. As the trail turns southeast, you will have a brief view upstream to the dam.

The gravel trail ends at 1.95 miles, at a gate signed 1.4 MILES TO FUEL BREAK ROAD AND CULVERT TRAIL. Follow the paved road as it turns to the left and begins to drop to the dam site and Lake Clementine. In 0.3 miles, a dirt footpath leaves the road and descends left. Those who want a very close look at the dam should take this short spur, which leads to the exact point at which the dam is anchored to the rock of the canyon wall. Along the way to this spot, notice the informal use-trail that descends to the river.

For a tamer look at the dam from a lakeside vantage point, continue along the paved road, turn left into the day-use parking lot, and descend to the lake level.

Retracing your steps will allow you to look for wildlife along the canyonside and flowers along the riverside. There is a long list of both, but you will be able to spot plenty of turkey vultures, squirrels, signs of coyotes, California quails, and scrub jays, along with turkeys and red-tailed hawks. Springtime brings a riot of color in this area, with Indian paintbrush, California poppy, lupine, and larkspur among the many flowers. Your hour-long return to the car will be a relaxing walk in one of the foothills' finest hiking regions.

■ TO THE TRAILHEAD

Drive 25 miles on Interstate 80 East to Auburn. Take the Elm Avenue exit and turn left at the traffic light. At the bottom of the hill, turn left at the High Street signal. From the railroad track overpass, a block ahead of you, drive 2.2 miles downhill on CA 49. Stay straight as it becomes Old Foresthill Road another 0.3 miles, crossing the bridge to find parking along the road. (You will pass the CA 49 turnoff, which goes east toward Cool and Georgetown.) Parking is allowed on both sides of the road. If you do need to park far from this spot, the trailhead is on the east side of the confluence.

13 Confluence Trail

■ OVERVIEW

LENGTH: 3.5 miles	**ACCESS:** No fees or permits
CONFIGURATION: Out-and-back	**MAPS:** USGS Auburn
WATER REQUIRED: 1 liter	**FACILITIES:** Pit toilet at the trailhead
SCENERY: Spectacular panorama of the Middle Fork of the American River	**WHEELCHAIR TRAVERSABLE:** No
	DRIVING DISTANCE: 28 miles
EXPOSURE: Exposed south-facing slope, with some trailside shade	**SPECIAL COMMENTS:** Information kiosks and pit toilets are located at the trailhead on the west side of Old Foresthill Road, and 200 feet west of the Old Foresthill Bridge on the north side of the road.
TRAFFIC: This is a popular hiking and mountain-biking trail.	
TRAIL SURFACE: Dirt and rock	
HIKING TIME: 1.5–2 hours	
SEASON: Year-round, sunrise–sunset	

■ SNAPSHOT

A short, gradual climb above the Middle Fork of the American River provides more than exercise. Hikers will be treated to panoramic, upriver views of the Middle Fork, overlooking placer mining and quarrying operations as they were left more than 100 years ago.

■ CLOSE-UP

The shaded trailhead is below the parking area on the west side of Old Foresthill Road. To reach it, descend from the parking area to the information kiosk and pit toilet. As you walk down toward the river, imagine cooling your feet at the river's edge after your hike.

Begin by walking south along the trail, directly toward the river. The first 500 feet make a sweeping curve from south to east. As you head away from the confluence, the trail begins an easy but steady uphill climb along a singletrack.

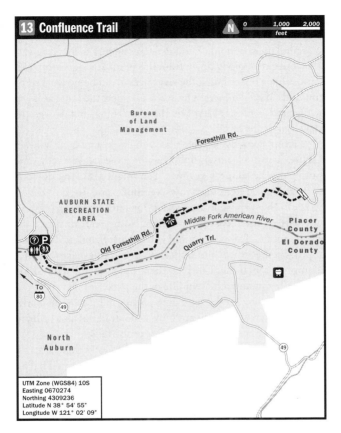

13 Confluence Trail

N   0   1,000   2,000
feet

Bureau
of Land
Management

Foresthill Rd.

AUBURN STATE
RECREATION
AREA

Old Foresthill Rd.

Middle Fork American River

Quarry Trl.

Placer
County

El Dorado
County

To
80

49

North
Auburn

49

UTM Zone (WGS84) 10S
Easting 0670274
Northing 4309236
Latitude N 38° 54' 55"
Longitude W 121° 02' 09"

The trail is sparsely shaded by foothill pine and cool manzanita. The pines can be recognized by their large (six- to teninch) globe-shaped cones, which are heavily armored with curved one-inch hooks at the ends of their scales—oddly overprotected and showy in comparison to the sparse, uneven growth of the tree itself.

Look to the south side of the middle fork, where the Quarry Trail runs parallel past Louisiana Bar, Warner's Ravine, New York

Bar, Murderer's Bar, Mammoth Bar, Murderer's Gulch, Texas Bar, Hoosier Bar, and on. The placer miners named these spots to remind them of home, and the names endure to this day.

Imagine looking down from this point at long, wood-and-canvas sluice boxes lining the river below and being worked by hundreds of gold miners. The scene is largely the same as it was in the mid–19th century, but the only thing that moves the rocks now is the river.

Keep your eyes peeled as you look across at Warner Ravine. The trail closely follows along the canyon side, and footing can be slippery at times. You might also look down at the trail and see signs of coyotes, raccoons, and dogs.

On this exposed slope watch for rattlesnakes, an important part of this ecosystem, seeking some warmth from the afternoon sun. They are shy and will not attack unless disturbed or provoked. Respect and walk away from rattlesnakes. Do not attempt to touch them or pick them up! It is unlawful to kill rattlesnakes or any other wildlife in the park.

Depending on the time of day, sun can be an issue. Early-morning hikers will enjoy not only a cool trail but also brilliant shows of light and shadow on the opposite hills.

The vehicular Old Foresthill Road follows this path as it rounds the mountain. Although the road is close, you'll have a hard time hearing any traffic. The trail surface changes from dirt and rock to old, broken pavement.

The hillsides here are exposed and lack the abundance of mosses seen on the North Fork trail. However, the mosses and ferns are replaced on this slope by chaparral flora, which now includes many nonnative grasses and flowers.

After about 0.75 miles, your singletrack trail becomes a FWD trail (or fire-suppression trail) that long ago saw its last vehicle. As the path turns east, pause to admire the view upriver from New York Bar below you to Murderer's Bar.

The Mammoth Bar area is reserved on specific days for off-highway-vehicle (OHV) users. Check with the park for the seasonal schedule by calling (530) 885-4527. Established OHV trails may be hiked when not reserved for OHV users.

After 1.75 miles, the trail ends at a gate signed TRAIL #107—EAST GATE and CONFLUENCE TRAIL. Retrace your steps to the trailhead. As you approach the confluence, the refreshing sounds of water will welcome you back.

■ MORE FUN

The Confluence Trail is well known to mountain biking enthusiasts. Auburn State Recreation Area (ASRA) has hundreds of miles of multiuse trails shared among equestrians, bikers, and hikers. Lake Clementine Trail and Quarry Road Trail in the Confluence area are well-regarded bike trails. The Olmstead Loop Trail in Cool was named in honor of a local bike shop owner and is a favorite among mountain bikers.

■ TO THE TRAILHEAD

Take Interstate 80 East 24 miles to the city of Auburn, then take the Elm Avenue exit and turn left at the traffic light. At the bottom of the hill, turn left at the High Street signal. From the railroad track overpass a block ahead of you, drive downhill on CA 49 2.2 miles where it becomes Old Foresthill Road, which you will stay on another 0.3 miles, crossing the bridge to find parking along the road. (You will pass the CA 49 turnoff, which goes east toward Cool and Georgetown.) Parking is allowed on both sides of the road.

■ OVERVIEW

LENGTH: 5.2 miles	**HIKING TIME:** 3 hours
CONFIGURATION: Out-and-back with loops	**SEASON:** Year-round
	ACCESS: No fees or permits
WATER REQUIRED: 2 liters	**MAPS:** USGS Auburn
SCENERY: Foothill woodland; views of North Fork of the American River, diversion tunnel, and Auburn Dam site	**WHEELCHAIR TRAVERSABLE:** No
	FACILITIES: None
EXPOSURE: In and out of shade	**DRIVING DISTANCE:** 26 miles
TRAFFIC: This is a multiuse trail that is regularly used by local residents.	**SPECIAL COMMENTS:** Heed the mountain-lion, rattlesnake, and poison-oak warnings.
TRAIL SURFACE: Dirt and duff, rock	

■ SNAPSHOT

You can hike in the Auburn State Recreation Area (ASRA) today on trails that were developed by California natives and pioneers. And the reason you can hike—rather than swim over—them is that the Auburn Dam wasn't built. This reminder of what could have been lost "if" may increase your appetite to see what is over the next hill.

■ CLOSE-UP

With more than 70 miles of hiking, biking, and horse-riding trails, the Auburn State Recreation Area is a gift for outdoors enthusiasts whose interests vary from fly fishing to gold panning. Twenty miles of the North Fork and Middle Fork of the American River are covered by ASRA, which is governed by the California State Parks for the U.S. Bureau of Reclamation.

The Robie Point Firebreak Trail guides the hiker through an area filled with the history of what once was, what is, and what was once to be. Heading downhill from the trailhead on

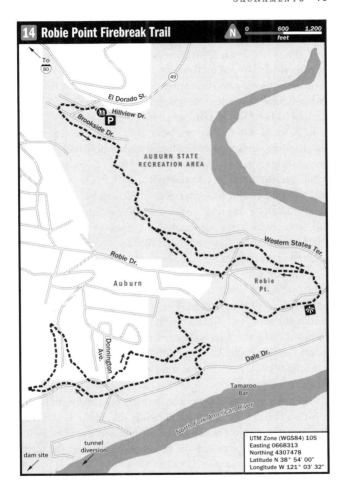

broken asphalt, look left and you will see the foundation of a hillside homestead just below the trail, which you should take to the right. Your wide path is bounded by lupine, buckeye, and rose. Ignore an old road to the right. Head past the blackberries and meander along the grassy trail. Within 0.25 miles, the sounds of the road diminish as you enter and exit a ravine.

The wide dirt trail heads generally southeast and is occasionally shaded by oak on the hillside above. At about 0.4 miles, turn back toward the confluence for a good view of the Foresthill Bridge, the pylons of which were to be completely submerged by the Auburn Dam reservoir.

A small dirt trail enters your path from the left at 0.7 miles, where you continue heading straight uphill. When a sign says AMERICAN DISCOVERY TRAIL—MILE 2, indicating an uphill track to the right, take the trail to the left. On your return, you will descend to this intersection from Robie Point. Turn around and look down to see the old road cuts and fills of hand-laid stone, which accommodated the track of the Mountain Quarries Railroad. Two of these fills are visible before you reach the point where the ponderosa pines lean over the trail.

As you make your way around the hillside below Robie Point, whiteleaf manzanita will shade you and Indian paintbrush will color the trailside. The path joining yours from the right is the trail you will take on the return to ascend to Robie Point. Shortly, the trail splits, with the Western States Trail (WST) heading right. The only difference is a few feet of elevation: the WST is more level and takes you to the same spot as the other one.

Turkey vultures hang out at the vista point beneath Robie Point waiting for the air to warm before taking the leap. From that spot, the entire Auburn Dam construction site comes into view to reveal the terracing, the diversion tunnel, and the western keyway for the dam itself.

The 0.5-mile-long diversion tunnel does not look 30 feet in diameter from this height. It was opened to redirect the waters of the North Fork to allow construction of the dam, which began in the dry riverbed to the right of the tunnel. In 1978 extensive seismic studies revealed the risk to the dam as it was then designed. By the late 1980s, the dam project had been stalled by additional design concerns. The project was later abandoned due to funding shortfalls. The original riverbed is now being restored, as are the surrounding hillsides and terraces.

Descend, stay on the WST, and ignore trails that enter or leave it. At a distinct fork in the trail, the WST heads right and past a green gate. You will return through this gate, but for now take the left trail, making a U-turn downhill. The trail is rocky and rutted, but there are good views as you switchback a few times along here. At another obvious intersection, you can take the trail that drops about 400 feet to Tamaroo Bar's rocky beach. However, your route takes the uphill trail to the right toward the telephone poles.

Just past the beginning of the power lines, at about 2.4 miles along, you will encounter a TRAIL CLOSED sign. Just as well, since the trail shortly becomes a paved road. The trail to the right, heading steeply uphill, looks enticing: follow it.

After a sweat-inducing huff-and-puff hill climb, you enter the cooling shade of a ravine-bound stream. Markers indicate that this is the WST and riders have only 1 mile to go to the finish. Wendell T. Robie was the founder of the Western States "100 Miles–One Day" Trail Ride, and it is in his memory that many trails have been named.

Pass the blackberries along this singletrack running through the shade and follow its WST markers to the green gate you eschewed earlier. Now a left turn takes you back the way you came.

When the trail splits after the vista point, take the left fork to go uphill to Robie Point. The trail comes out next to Gate 135, Robie Point to Murphy's Gate–Highway 49, which is on one side of a cul-de-sac; opposite it are Gates 133, Robie Point to Marion Way, and 134, Robie Point to WST. Walk down the trail past Gate 135 to rejoin the doubletrack you traveled earlier.

Large, yellow-and-black western tiger swallowtail butterflies will outpace you down the trail as they head for the big cone-shaped collection of flowers gracing branches of California buckeye. Other butterflies are also attracted to these sweet-smelling bouquets: Amusingly, the little gray Hairstreaks and California sisters seem to demand aerial battles before they will permit intruders to drink up the nectar.

On your way back to the trailhead, fragrances are brought to you by Chinese houses, lupine, buckeye, California rose, and larkspur. A final plunge into the ravine will cool you off before the short climb to the trailhead.

■ TO THE TRAILHEAD

From the junction of Interstate 80 East and Capital City Freeway, drive 25 miles to the Elm Street exit in Auburn. Turn left at the traffic light onto Elm Street. At the bottom of the hill turn left again, onto High Street. Pass beneath the Southern Pacific Railroad trestle as you continue downhill on CA 49. Look for the Auburn State Recreation Area sign on the right. The trailhead is 0.2 miles after that sign, also on the right. The number of horseshoes attached to the oak distinguishes this large lot. Your trailhead is at the green gate marked gate 130— MURPHY'S GATE TO ROBIE POINT.

15 Hardrock Trail

■ OVERVIEW

LENGTH: 4.2 miles	**SEASON:** Year-round, sunrise–sunset
CONFIGURATION: Connected loops	**ACCESS:** $6 fee at visitor center
WATER REQUIRED: 1 liter	**MAPS:** USGS Grass Valley; local trail map available in visitor center
SCENERY: Foothill woodland, historic mining relics and buildings	
	FACILITIES: Parking at Penn Gate is free; restrooms at visitor center
EXPOSURE: Mostly shaded	
TRAFFIC: Moderate	**WHEELCHAIR TRAVERSABLE:** No
TRAIL SURFACE: Dirt and duff, gravel and sand	**DRIVING DISTANCE:** 48 miles
	SPECIAL COMMENTS: Hazardous-waste cleanup has temporarily closed some portions of the trails.
HIKING TIME: 2 hours	

■ SNAPSHOT

The Hardrock Trail loops around the 800-acre Empire Mine State Historic Park, guiding hikers through the relics of the region's richest gold-mining area. Additional loops adjoin this trail, allowing hikers to create their own routes.

■ CLOSE-UP

Hardrock mining came to Nevada County in 1850 when George Knight discovered gold—literally a mountain of it. The Mother Lode he unearthed not only was one of the richest gold deposits in the world but also became the descriptive name for the entire region. More than half of California's gold production came from the mines in this area, with the Empire Mine and the North Star Mine yielding the greatest share of riches.

The Hardrock Trail begins at Penn Gate, which is close to the old Pennsylvania Mine site. The Pennsylvania Mine was one of many dotting the park grounds. In the 1850s, mine shafts were blasted, drilled, and dug in every direction to extract gold-bearing ore for further processing. Ore was crushed to sand by

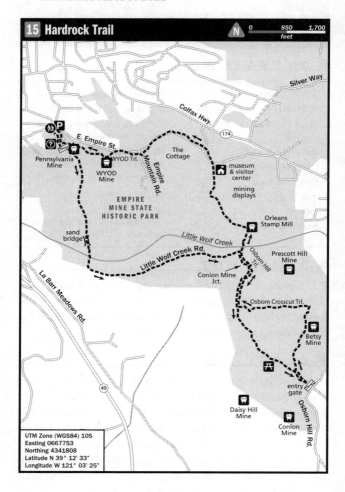

15 Hardrock Trail

N   0   850   1,700
                 feet

Silver Way

Colfax Hwy.

174

E. Empire St.

WYOD Trl.

The Cottage

museum & visitor center

Pennsylvania Mine

WYOD Mine

mining displays

EMPIRE MINE STATE HISTORIC PARK

Empire Mountain Rd.

Orleans Stamp Mill

sand bridge

Little Wolf Creek

Prescott Hill Mine

Little Wolf Creek Rd.

Osborn Hill Trl.

Conlon Mine Jct.

La Barr Meadows Rd.

Osborn Crosscut Trl.

Betsy Mine

entry gate

49

Daisy Hill Mine

Conlon Mine

Osborn Hill Rd.

UTM Zone (WGS84) 10S
Easting 0667753
Northing 4341808
Latitude N 39° 12' 33"
Longitude W 121° 03' 25"

the numerous and noisy stamp mills. The resulting ore dust was treated with chemicals—the most hazardous of which were mercury and cyanide—to capture the gold. Your trail passes by the stamp mills, tailings piles, and slurry ponds, which are currently being cleaned up so the area can be reclaimed by nature.

An information kiosk at the trailhead displays a map giving an overview of the trails. It also houses a very active colony of carpenter bees, which encourages speed-reading. It is best to pick up a current trails guide from the visitor center. Heed the warnings about both rattlesnakes and mountain lions.

The interpretive signs along the trail help visitors appreciate the area's history. What may look like a pile of useless rock turns out to be, well, a pile of useless rock that was placed there on purpose by individual miners toiling in the Work Your Own Diggins Mine. Operated somewhat like a time-share scheme, the mine was finally abandoned in 1912.

A chain-link fence on your left borders the trail as you walk south toward Little Wolf Creek. Keep close to the fence and cross over the sand dam to the left. Then cross a small footbridge over the creek before turning east on Little Wolf Creek Road. Under shade of ponderosa pine and a stand of big leaf maple, walk leisurely uphill to travel above the creek to your left.

After walking east 1 mile, you encounter a junction with the Osborn Loop Trail and the Union Hills trails. With the promise of several abandoned mines, turn right, and then at the next junction follow the right-hand fork uphill. This is the apex of the Osborn Hill Loop when all the trails are open. Hazardous waste cleanup is ongoing, and trails may be rerouted.

The next south-bearing section of trail is exposed, as it gains about 200 feet over the next half mile. Pass the Daisy Hill Mine on the right. For observant hikers, there is a fenced-off mine shaft to the left. Pass under the power lines and note the trail beneath it. The described hike will later return you to this point.

Just in time for a brief water break, you will find a picnic table shaded by pine and fir. Despite the park-service sign, there is no scenic lookout but rather a trail downhill to Daisy Hill Mine. If you want to take this side trip, it is only 0.25 miles to the site, but dense whiteleaf manzanita makes it difficult to find the actual site remains. If you hit the fence, turn back 100 feet for the mine site. Stay on the main trail to continue toward Conlon Mine, which is just 500 feet past the next intersection.

There is a gate adjacent to the mine site that allows access from Osborn Hill Road and Comet Lane.

When you return to the junction from the Conlon Mine site (which may be fenced off for cleanup), turn right on the Osborn Loop Trail, heading south in the direction of the Prescott Hill Mine and the Hardrock Trail. On the way, you will pass the trail to the Betsy Mine on your right. A fence at Osborn Hill Road will turn you around if you explore this side trail.

An area closure around the Prescott Hill Mine abbreviates the Osborn Hill Loop. So turn to the west when you reach the Osborn Crosscut Trail (underneath the power lines) until you zigzag to the left and right at the Power Line Trail. This is an unpleasant hilly stretch of cruddy trail that is very exposed to the sun. You will recognize the point you passed earlier and you will turn right to head north, back toward the Hardrock Trail.

Follow the trail signs toward an easily crossed Little Wolf Creek. At the top of the brief uphill, the trail turns left to pass by the foundations of the Orleans Stamp Mill. Your trail continues to the back of the visitor center. The Hardrock Trail continues on East Empire Street along the stone wall in front of the Bourne mansion. Penn Gate is only 0.5 miles ahead.

Before you reach your destination, you will pass the Mule Corral; here mules awaited their descent into the mines, where they worked out their lives and birthed generations of new stock. You will again walk through the Pennsylvania Mine remains as the trailhead comes into view.

■ TO THE TRAILHEAD

From Interstate 80 East and the Capital City freeway, drive 24 miles east to Auburn. Take the CA 49 exit northbound to Grass Valley. Drive about 22 miles to the Empire Street exit and turn right onto West Empire Street. Cross South Auburn Street and continue 0.3 miles on East Empire Street to the Penn Gate trailhead parking area on the right.

OVERVIEW

LENGTH: 4.6 miles (West Trail only)	**WHEELCHAIR TRAVERSABLE:** Yes; all facilities are accessible.
CONFIGURATION: Out-and-back	
SCENERY: Foothill forest, canyon overlooks	**FACILITIES:** Restrooms at trailhead and 2 spots along the trail; no water available
EXPOSURE: Always shaded	
TRAFFIC: Moderate	**DRIVING DISTANCE:** 57 miles
TRAIL SURFACE: Leaf-covered duff and dirt	**SPECIAL COMMENTS:** This is the nation's first wheelchair-accessible wilderness trail. Groups may take a docent-guided tour by calling (530) 272-0298. The East Branch is temporarily closed for extensive trail maintenance and flume reconstruction. Fortunately, of the two branches, the West Branch is the more scenic.
HIKING TIME: 1–3 hours	
SEASON: Year-round	
ACCESS: No fees or permits	
MAPS: USGS Nevada City; local trail map available at Tahoe NF Ranger Station on CA 49	

SNAPSHOT

Just ten minutes from Nevada City, this pleasant hike makes use of the first wheelchair-accessible wilderness trail in the United States. The builders created the path from the remains of an abandoned mining and irrigation canal originally built in 1854. The level grade makes it ideal for hikers of all ages and abilities. Interpretive and identifying signs highlight the diversity of flora along the trail. A sharp eye will spot a California newt among the trail duff (and the sharp hiker will not touch it—its slimy coating is toxic). The cascades at Rush Creek, which has a superior ramp-access system, are the glamour spot on this route.

CLOSE-UP

Gold Country trails certainly offer foothill hikers some diverse and lush flora. The trail itself runs along a mining relic: In 1854

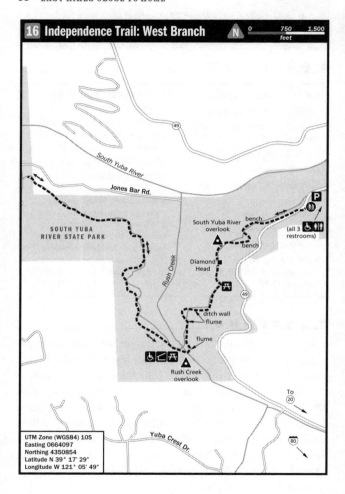

16 Independence Trail: West Branch

N 0   750   1,500
        feet

South Yuba River

Jones Bar Rd.

SOUTH YUBA
RIVER STATE PARK

Rush Creek

South Yuba River
overlook

Diamond
Head

bench

bench

(all 3
restrooms)

ditch wall
flume

flume

Rush Creek
overlook

To
(20)

(80)

Yuba Crest Dr.

UTM Zone (WGS84) 10S
Easting 0664097
Northing 4350854
Latitude N 39° 17' 29"
Longitude W 121° 05' 49"

the Excelsior Mining and Canal Company constructed the
Excelsior Ditch to transport water from the South Yuba River
17 miles to join another canal near the present-day Lake Wild-
wood dam. This nearly level ditch and the maintenance trail
beside it are now your route.

The East and West branches share a common trailhead. Your trail, the West Branch, is the more scenic of the two. Signs on the information board will direct you if you forgot your compass.

You almost immediately enter a short tunnel to pass safely underneath CA 49. Signs there inform hikers that leashed dogs are permitted on the trail, but bicycles, motorcycles, camping, and fires are not. Beware of the poison oak.

The reinforced fence borders this initial stretch, separating hikers from exposed, steep hillsides. The trail has three distinct segments, which you will notice from the outset. In the first 0.1 mile, you will see the stone wall (probably covered with moss and lichen), which is the original wall of the ditch. Adjacent to and slightly above the ditch path is the path for the ditch tenders who monitored the water flow and made repairs. The most unusual features along the path are the flumes—wooden troughs standing on trestles—which carried the water across ravines and other streams.

A bench fashioned from a large tree trunk sits next to the first bridge at the 0.2-mile point. Within another 50 feet, Jones Bar Trail leads off to the north. Stay left on Independence Trail. Notice the incense cedar mixed in with Pacific madrone as you make your way down to the next bridge and another log bench.

Look closely for the interpretive signs for the towering ponderosa pine, the canyon live oak, and Kellogg black oak, which happen to surround the excellent South Yuba River Overlook, which you will reach after 0.4 miles. Here is a nice shelter in case of sudden showers.

As you walk 500 feet on, notice the deerbrush and manzanita bushes shading you from even the low morning sun. A series of ramps lead you to Diamond Head—a class-A outhouse at the 0.5-mile point in your hike.

You will have the sensation of descending into the canyon, but it is an illusion caused by CA 49 climbing up the hill as the trail stays level. As the sound of cars falls away, you will notice more and more ferns, mosses, and lichens along the rock walls. Amble 500 feet more and you will encounter an outhouse and a picnic table. So far you have traveled 0.6 miles.

Look up at the Douglas fir now towering over you and the bigleaf maple shading you when its leaves are full. In the next few hundred feet, you are going to notice the air becoming cooler where moist, moss-covered rocks surround you. These rocks remain as they were when laid here more than 150 years ago. Although reconstructed, Flumes 26 and 27 are identical in design to the water-carrying structures of the gold-rush days. By the time you reach Flume 27 you will have walked just about a mile.

Your south-facing trail still gets plenty of shade from the surrounding manzanita and may be muddy in some spots along here. If you look carefully, you will probably spot a California newt. The male newt may puff himself up, showing his reddish abdomen; but his defense is in his skin, which has a coating toxic to humans. Shoot a photo and leave the newt alone.

California buckeyes line the path here as you come upon another small shelter allowing a shaded overlook to the South Yuba River below. The best site is still ahead about 500 feet, where you will come upon Flume 28. Its horseshoe shape illustrates exactly how the ditch builders shortcut most ravines by building a trestle with a flume atop it.

This flume is special in that it allows easy access to the pool at the base of the cascades of Rush Creek. This is truly an idyllic spot. In winter the ice clings to the rocks surrounding the pond, and in the spring, water shoots with a roar across the rocks these ramps overlook. Benches, a shelter, wide shallow ramps, and a tree-shaded pool. Spectacular.

As you leave Rush Creek the trail turns north, traveling along the opposite side of the ravine. If you're ready for a snack, picnic tables are about 200 steps ahead. Ramps lead to the tables and to an outhouse at the end of the platform.

The trail ends at Jones Bar Road, an obvious turnaround spot. Retrace your steps to the trailhead or drop down to Jones Bar and the beaches along the river.

Independence Trail: East Branch

By mid-summer 2008, flume reconstruction was complete and the East branch of the Independence Trail was reopened. From the same trailhead as the West branch, your northeasterly route along the Excelsior Ditch leads you 2.2 miles to the Miner's Tunnel Overlook close to Hoyt Crossing.

The trail leads you under Tunnel Rock, across carefully refurbished flumes on their trestles which span ravines and cling to granite outcrops, over cascading Augustini Creek, to your destination 2.2 miles from the trailhead. On your return, enjoy a shaded picnic at the table next to the spring which feeds Augustini Creek.

TOTAL HIKING TIME: 2.5 hours

■ TO THE TRAILHEAD

From the junction of Interstate 80 with the Capitol City Freeway, drive 24 miles east on I-80 to Auburn. Exit at CA 49 and drive 27 miles north to Nevada City, then turn left—following CA 49—at the split with CA 20. Immediately to your right is the Tahoe National Forest ranger station, where you can obtain additional trail information and a simple map. The trailhead is 6.2 miles past the ranger station. A parking area with enough room for a dozen cars is on the right side of CA 49, in front of the trailhead and restrooms.

17 Buttermilk Bend Trail

■ OVERVIEW

LENGTH: 2.5 miles

CONFIGURATION: Out-and-back

WATER REQUIRED: 0.5 liters

SCENERY: Spectacular views of the South Yuba River

EXPOSURE: Partially shaded trail with exposed areas

TRAFFIC: Moderate

TRAIL SURFACE: Dirt and rock

HIKING TIME: 1.5 hours

SEASON: Year-round; parking sunrise–sunset

ACCESS: No fees or permits

MAPS: USGS French Corral

WHEELCHAIR TRAVERSABLE: No

FACILITIES: Toilets in parking area and at nearby visitor center

DRIVING DISTANCE: 62.5 miles

SPECIAL COMMENTS: For more information about the South Yuba River State Park, see www.ncgold.com/Museums_Parks.syrp. If you want more exercise and a different view of the river, take the Point Defiance Trail 1 mile to Englebright Lake and return. The Point Defiance Trail begins across the road and about 100 yards down at a signed trailhead adjacent to the covered bridge.

■ SNAPSHOT

Prepare for extraordinary views of the South Yuba River from rock benches along this easy trail. Here, the riparian zone holds somewhat closely to the river's edge, quickly transitioning to a foothill woodland zone upslope. The result is a transition zone that boasts the best of both zones. The abundance of flowers and trees along this short, friendly trail makes this a favorite foothill hike for all ages.

■ CLOSE-UP

Starting your trip from the second parking lot is easiest, but whether you park here or back across the river next to the bridge, take time to cross the Bridgeport Bridge.

The Bridgeport Bridge has the distinction of being the longest single-span covered bridge in America. Built in 1862, it

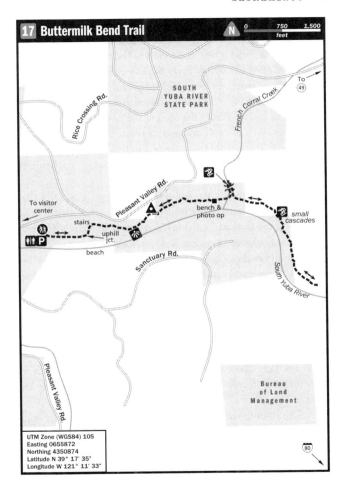

is one of only ten covered bridges left in California. Made from Douglas fir and covered with sugar-pine shingles, the bridge's double-truss and hoop construction is unique. The only other bridge of its design was built in New York. Information in the visitor center will explain how this bridge's architecture is responsible for its strength, durability, and beauty.

Your trailhead is near the toilets in the north parking lot. If you parked here, the trail is obvious. However, if you parked next to the visitor center, traverse the bridge and turn right onto the path leading past the picnic table and information sign, then walk through the gate and cross the road to the north lot.

Signs warn of rattlesnakes and mountain lions along this trail. These are sensible warnings for this area, despite this being such an easy trail. Colorful poison oak is particularly common along spots of this trail as well.

The trail initially rises above the river so gradually that you might miss some of the interpretive signs that identify the flora along the trail and hillsides. Beginning in March, California poppies, popcorn flowers, larkspurs, shooting stars, fiddlenecks, and blue dicks splash across the slopes above and below you and at every seep and spring coming in from your left. Stop frequently to read about them. Smell them endlessly. But leave them to grow, as the park requests. The more seeds that fall, the more flowers will grow.

The trail you are on is about 75 yards below an alternate trailhead that starts in the original flume dug in the hillside in 1877. Looking above the trail to the left, you may see some of those original flume works. Your trail will join with that leg shortly.

The smooth wire fence to your right is there to steady your nerves because the trail runs above the river along an abrupt precipice. As you begin to notice the enormous cobble littering the river in front of you, the trail will ascend a short hill. At the top of this rise, a side trail to the right descends to the river.

Follow the trail uphill to the left, past the miner's lettuce and flowering redbud. Directly after this junction, you should be able to see some stairs ahead of you. Get ready for a quick elevation gain—these 35 stairs pop you up to some switchbacks on an exposed slope. The dirt path is quite well defined now and will soon be joined from the left by the upper trail. You are now in the original flume and the trail will remain level to its end.

When you can distinctly hear the river, just as the trail turns northeast, you will have a great view of the pools and beach below. In another 20 steps, there will be a bench cut into the rock. Purple spring vetch, orange California poppy, and white canyon nemophila grow around you at this up-canyon viewpoint.

Another side trail, with stairs at the top, leads down to the river. Your path continues northeast, where you will find a stone bench right at the bend in the trail marked by the large foothill pine. The view overlooking the cascades is fantastic.

Continue eastward, with miniature lupine and bird's-foot fern lining the trail. A small ravine has been strengthened by some recent rockwork above and below the trail. Another vantage point—allowing you to see around Buttermilk Bend—is equipped with a stone bench. The cascades below make for a great photo.

After walking north for a few minutes, you will cross a bridge over the ravine at French Corral Creek. The bridge is wide and you can linger to watch the water cascading above and below the bridge. You can also head left after crossing the bridge to sit on the rocks and observe the streamside insect activity.

After crossing the bridge, make a U-turn to exit the ravine. Look back to the obvious stonework on the opposite side of the bridge, and now look next to you for similar formations. These are the abutments for the original flume that crossed the ravine.

As you leave the ravine, look for the deep purple of the zigzag larkspur, popcorn flower, and blue dick around the rock outcropping. The toyon has been trimmed back but still shades much of the trail. Blue oak and foothill pine also ensure a cool hike.

Depending on the season, you may be able to see some relics of the gold-mining era—other than your trail. This is reported to have been a mining area, and so large numbers of people were encamped right below your path. The stone fireplace, just about 50 feet below the trail, may indicate a dwelling more permanent than a tent—a home or a boarding house. The large metal pieces that look like monitor pipes are said to be sections of a hoist for moving rocks.

Just 1.25 miles ahead, the South Yuba River State Park ends. You can descend one of two trails that angle toward boulders as big as midsize cars. After exploring at the river, retrace your steps to the trailhead.

■ MORE FUN

The Kneebone Family Cemetery and the Bridgeport Barn are on the grounds of the nearby Bridgeport Visitor Center.

■ TO THE TRAILHEAD

From the junction of Interstate 80 East and the Capital City Freeway, drive approximately 24 miles east on I-80 to the CA 49 north exit in Auburn. Drive about 23 miles toward Grass Valley, and exit toward Marysville on CA 20. Head 7.5 miles on CA 20 to Pleasant Valley Road, then bear right and drive 7.7 miles to the Bridgeport Visitor Center. You can park in the lot on your left just past the large barn or continue across the bridge and park in the lot on your right, on the road, or directly in front of the trailhead, next to the toilets.